Sexuality, Curiosity, Fear, and the Arts

New Studies in Aesthetics

Robert Ginsberg
General Editor

Vol. 33

PETER LANG
New York • Washington, D.C./Baltimore • Bern
Frankfurt am Main • Berlin • Brussels • Vienna • Oxford

Milton D. Heifetz

Sexuality, Curiosity, Fear, and the Arts

Biology of Aesthetics

PETER LANG
New York • Washington, D.C./Baltimore • Bern
Frankfurt am Main • Berlin • Brussels • Vienna • Oxford

Library of Congress Cataloging-in-Publication Data

Heifetz, Milton D.
Sexuality, curiosity, fear, and the arts:
biology of aesthetics / Milton D. Heifetz.
p. cm. — (New studies in aesthetics; vol. 33)
Includes bibliographical references and index.
1. Aesthetics—Psychological aspects. I. Title. II. Series.
BH301.P78 H45 111′.85—dc21 00-062972
ISBN 0-8204-5231-9
ISSN 0893-6005

Die Deutsche Bibliothek-CIP-Einheitsaufnahme

Heifetz, Milton D.:
Sexuality, curiosity, fear, and the arts:
biology of aesthetics / Milton D. Heifetz.
–New York; Washington, D.C./Baltimore; Bern;
Frankfurt am Main; Berlin; Brussels; Vienna; Oxford: Lang.
(New studies in aesthetics; Vol. 33)
ISBN 0-8204-5231-9

The paper in this book meets the guidelines for permanence and durability
of the Committee on Production Guidelines for Book Longevity
of the Council of Library Resources.

Printed in the United States of America

To Betsy

Table of Contents

Acknowledgments

This work has been incubating over many years during which time my wife, Betsy, and our four children, Laurence, Daniel, Ronald, and Deborah have read, sometimes under protest, various versions of this manuscript, and have commented with enlightening perception and wisdom.

I have been very fortunate to have had the constructive criticisms of James S. Ackerman, Theodore Baker, Hilda Branch, J. Woodland Hastings, Harold Heifetz, Philip Isenberg, Jerome Kagan, Judd Marmor, and Pinchas Noy. Their comments and suggestions have been of immense value. I wish to express my appreciation to Manfred Clynes, Uri Haber-Schaim, Mark Lindley, Margarita Mazo, and Nigel Nettheim for their suggestions concerning the section on the relationship between minor mode music and melancholy. I also am thankful to Gerald Berlin for his critique of the chapter on the critic. My editor, Robert Ginsberg, portrayed a dedication that went beyond the call of duty.

I would also like to thank the following institutions for their permission to reprint from the following works:

> *Magdalen with the Smoking Flame*, circa 1640 Georges de la Tour, oil on canvas, 46 1/16 x 36 1/8 in. (117 x 91.76 cm). © 2000 Museum Associates/LACMA. Los Angeles County Museum of Art, Gift of The Ahmanson Foundation, reprinted with the permission of the publisher.

> *Woman with the Blue Veil*, 1923. Pablo Picasso, oil on canvas, 39 1/2. x 32 in. (100.33 x 81.28 cm). © 2000 Museum Associates/LACMA. Los Angeles County Museum of Art Mr. and Mrs. George Gard de Sylva Collection, reprinted with the permission of the publisher.

Woman with the Blue Veil, Pablo Picasso. © 2000 Estate of Pablo Picasso/Artists Rights Society (ARS), New York.

"The Term" by William Carlos Williams, from *Collected Poems: 1909 1939, Volume I*, copyright © 1938 by New Directions Publishing Corp. Reprinted by permission of New Directions Publishing Corp.

"The Term" by William Carlos Williams, from *Collected Poems: 1909–1939, Volume I*, copyright © 1938 Carcanet Press Limited. Reprinted by permission of 1938 Carcanet Press Limited.

Introduction

This work is intended to help clarify the biological under-pinnings of aesthetics and thereby lead to a better understanding of why we feel what we feel upon exposure to the arts. It does not pretend to be a comprehensive theory of aesthetics, nor does it explain the complex psychological convolutions that enable the human mind to sense the awesome and the beautiful, but it aims to clarify the foundation upon which that capability rests.

In the process of discussion I propose definitions of aesthetics, art, beauty, and the sublime. These definitions may soften the attitude of Mary Mothersill who believes that any "attempt to define art or beauty…is a mistake….Aesthetics is an intellectual wasteland…due to the lack of adequate definitions."[1]

"She is joined in this view by Morris Weitz who believes that "Aesthetic theory—all of it—is wrong in principle…," and who concludes that "aesthetic theory is a…vain attempt to define what cannot be defined, to state the necessary and sufficient properties of that which has no necessary and sufficient properties…."[2]

A fundamental issue concerning the relationship between a work of art and the perceiver is the role of emotion. Susanne K. Langer rejects the claim that art always evokes emotion. She states:

> the tacit assumption that what is expressed in art is always an emotion, when in fact it may be the mere feeling of vitality, energy or somnolence, or the sense of quietness, or of concentration, or any of the countless inward actions and conditions which are felt in the living fabric of mental life.[3]

Langer's concept appears nonsensical since the "mere feeling of vitality" and "sense of quietness" are biologically tied to emotion.

Her concept suggests a sharp division between the anatomical source of our emotion, the limbic system, the primitive portion of our brain, and the neocortex of the human brain. This contradicts biological fact and psychological understanding. To imply that these qualities exist independent of emotion seems extremely rash. Jean Piaget referred to this problem. He said:

> if one attempts to dichotomize the life of the mind into emotions and thoughts...nothing could be more false...affectivity and intelligence are indissociable and constitute the two complementary aspects of all human behavior.[4]

But Langer's phrase "mere feeling" deserves clarification. Sensations quite likely exist that do not automatically send impulses to the limbic system and therefore, at that moment, may be devoid of emotional content. Unlike complex feelings of vitality and quietness, they are sensations of pure cortical awareness, for example, awareness of a simple number, the "unaware awareness" of stepping off a curb, or the semiconscious awareness of objects in our peripheral vision as we drive along the highway.

Contrary to Langer, we might rather assume that a work that does not incite emotion cannot be art, while what incites emotion is not necessarily art.

Deryck Cooke strongly supports this position in relation to music:

> whatever else the mysterious art known as music may eventually be found to express, it is primarily and basically a language of the emotions, through which we directly experience the fundamental urges that move mankind, without the need of falsifying ideas and images—words or pictures.[5]

A.J. Ayer also strongly supported the idea that all aesthetic value judgements are expressions of emotion,[6] as did Clive Bell, who believed that "The starting-point for all systems of aesthetics must be the personal experience of a peculiar emotion."[7] Roger Fry joins this view. He states that "In the case of works of art the whole end and purpose is found in the exact quality of the emotional state."[8]

The assumption that art and emotion are always inter-twined will serve as the basis for the following discussion. Although much has been written on the subject in the psychoanalytic literature, as well as in philosophy, explanations concerning the fundamental emotional mechanisms underlying our reactions to the arts are still inconclusive.[9] The exact relationship between emotion and the arts has been difficult to clarify. My intention in this work is to clarify those mechanisms and thereby help establish a firmer foundation upon which discussions of art and the emotion it incites may rest. Edmund Burke referred to this approach: "A consideration of the rationale of our passions seems to me very necessary for all who would affect them upon solid and sure principles."[10]

To better understand the art-emotion relationship necessitates an understanding of what we mean by emotion. Therefore, the first chapter discusses the origin of human emotion, its anatomical and psychological foundation, fundamental emotional patterns and their function, and the effect of learning on emotion.

The second chapter examines the basic psychological mechanisms that lead to pleasure. The word "pleasure," encountered throughout this work, should be understood as a generic term that includes all desirable feelings: feelings associated with sensuality, exposure to music, gratification, feelings of comfort, and feelings of relief from discomfort. These feelings of pleasure are quite unlike each other.[11] The pleasure of taste is unlike the pleasure obtained from music or sexuality.

Chapter three explores the most fundamental relationships between art and emotion. This leads to a definition of aesthetics in Chapter four that is followed by a definition of art in Chapter five. Chapter six discusses the concepts of beauty, ugly, and the sublime in an attempt to define their boundaries. Chapter seven explains the influence of biology on the appreciation or lack of appreciation of non-objective art.

The subsequent three chapters, which may be considered as Part two, are not directly related to evolutionary biological influences, but they are included since I believe them to be psychologically pertinent in our relationship to the arts and the artist. Chapter eight discusses the significance of the aesthetic "attitude" and its potential impact upon observance of the commonplace. Chapter nine concerns the obligations engendered within the artist-society relationship. This is followed by a discussion of the function of the Critic in Chapter ten.

This work is not intended to grade, measure, compare, or assess the relative value of any art form or the relative significance of works of art within a given art form. My primary intent is to clarify the foundation upon which aesthetics rests and secondly to set the parameters that may determine whether a work has aesthetic significance and is therefore a work of art. Comparative studies of different works of art, whether in music, painting, dance, architecture, or other art forms, rightfully belong as subjects of inquiry within the superstructure of aesthetics rather than to its foundation.

Chapter One

The Anatomy of Human Emotion

The complexities of emotion are beyond the scope of this work, but we can grasp its basic nature if we appreciate some of the evolutionary aspects leading to the formation of the human brain, its relationship to the primitive emotions that are common to all mammals, and the remarkable persistence of these primitive feeling states in the brain of humans.

The fundamental biological forces, the remarkable physics and chemistry that drive a human animal are essentially the same forces that drive a seedling to penetrate and explode the overlying rock on its way to reach sunlight. These awesome forces, that became manifest with the beginning of living chemistry, continue their presence and thrust toward life whether it be within the most primitive single-cell animal or plant or within the most sophisticated human being.

As animal life developed, each more advanced creature received from its predecessor genetically determined forces and behavior patterns. These patterns were, and still are, directed toward two fundamental evolutionary principles: to preserve the self and to preserve the species.

The drives to preserve the self and to perpetuate the species depend upon feeling states that either help alert the animal to environmental conditions, such as danger, so that it may respond appropriately, or act as motivating forces to awaken and animate behavior patterns leading toward procreation. These primitive feeling states are the precursors of human emotion.

James Papez, a pioneer in understanding the mechanism of emotion, describes it this way:

> 'emotion' as commonly used implies two conditions: a way of acting and a way of feeling. The former is designated as emotional expression; the latter, as emotional experience or subjective feeling…emotional expression depends on the integrative action of the hypothalamus rather than on that of the dorsal thalamus or cortex, since it may occur when the cerebral hemispheres and the dorsal thalamus are totally removed. For subjective emotional experience, however, the participation of the cortex is essential. Emotional expression and emotional experience may in the human subject be dissociated phenomena.[1]

The animalistic feelings, the "primitive emotions," associated with self-preservation patterns are generally unpleasant. They are primarily fear, nausea, hunger, apprehension, and tension; feelings basically agitative and undesirable. Their undesirable nature impels the animal to avoid or nullify forces that produce such reactions and threaten life. The distress of hunger and the resultant aggressive pattern of seeking food, like the patterns of defense as a reaction to life's threats, reflects this dynamic. If these feelings were pleasurable and therefore desirable, they would serve to endanger rather than to protect life. Natural selection would tend to eliminate individuals with such undesirable tendencies.

The feelings associated with species-preservation as sensuality, cuddling, caressing, and affection, are primarily gratifying and pleasurable in character and as such predispose to foster activities that would ensure and enhance the continuation of the species.

Homo sapiens have developed the ability to develop secondary pleasurable effects from the unpleasant feelings associated with self preservation. An example is that as the displeasure of hunger is negated the secondary effect of producing pleasure through the sensations of taste and smell may develop. This eventually leads to the aesthetics of fine food.

Anatomical Aspects

The brain of reptiles and lower mammals has a thin layer of cells, the cortex, that partially or completely covers the main mass of the brain, termed the limbic system or limbic lobe. The cortex serves primarily to sense external input and to effect motor function.

The cortex of lower animals is not adequate for significant reasoning processes. Lower vertebrates therefore function primarily, although not totally, in a non-reasoning manner. They act and react almost entirely reflexively, instinctively, according to inherited feeling states and behavior patterns under control of the limbic system.

In the evolutionary process toward human beings, this thin primitive cortex slowly thickened and expanded to reach its culmination in the massive new cortex (neocortex) of Homo sapiens. The formation of the neocortex produced a marked increase in surface area. This allowed for the development of innumerable association pathways. The unique quality of this association network underlies a human being's ability to learn, imagine, create, control and expand primitive feeling states.

This remarkable expansion of the cortex has been referred to by C.J. Herrick as "One of the most dramatic cases of evolutionary transformation known to comparative anatomy."[2] What is remarkable in this development is that while the primitive cortex became quite large, the remainder of the primitive brain (its main mass containing the site of animalistic feelings), persisted and exists in the center of the human brain relatively unchanged. As a result, the primary animalistic feelings persist as the foundation upon which human emotion is built. Although some anatomic changes have taken place, the function of this "primitive brain" in human beings is basically the same as in lower mammals and is now referred to as the limbic system. This segment of the human brain integrates the mechanisms involved in self- and species-preservation. It is the anatomic center for human emotion.[3]

One of the more interesting anatomic changes that has taken place in the evolutionary process toward human beings concerns the intimate relationship between primitive animal behavior and the olfactory sense. This close relationship plays a major role in the feeding and mating habits of lower mammals. In human beings this anatomic relationship has slowly shifted away from olfaction to vision. This shift is reflected in the socio-sexual behavior of men and women during which eye contact, facial expression and body image play a major role.[4]

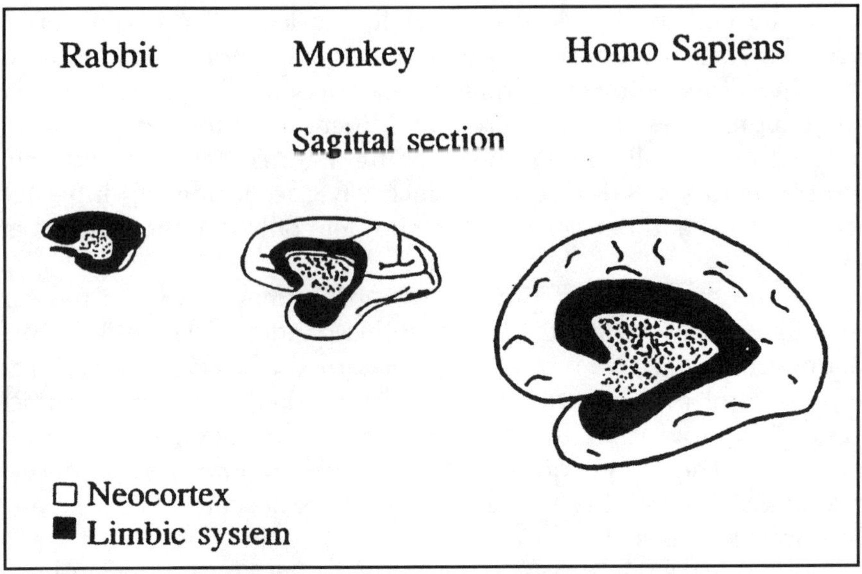

Figure 1: Relative Ratios between the Cortex and the Limbic System
Adapted from Paul MacLean, "New Findings Relevant to the Evolution of Psychosexual Functions of the Brain," in *Journal of Nervous and Mental Disease* (October 1962).

Despite extensive anatomic evolutionary changes, human emotion and behavior patterns are basically no different than those of a mouse, dog or a monkey, but unlike lower mammals this substrate has been significantly influenced by the growth of the overlying cortex.

George Mandler believes that the degree of plasticity of human beings, the complexity of emotional patterns and our psychological convolutions suggest that human emotions are not necessarily tied to basic animalistic impulses.[5]

I disagree with this evaluation. The remarkable plasticity and complexity of human emotion only reflects the ability of our neocortex to overtly ignore basic impulses, but that does not mean that our feelings have lost their ties to the primitive brain. For emotion to be aroused, the neural impulse received by the brain must be transmitted to the limbic system. I strongly doubt that emotion is ever a purely neocortical function.

Emotion is almost always associated with internal changes of the body. When emotion reaches a certain level of intensity, it is productive of physical changes such as facial flush, rapid heart beat and respiration, sweating, and dryness of the throat.[6]

Most studies of emotion concern themselves with the parameters of these physical changes since they are readily subject to measurements. Further attempts to define emotion were essentially ignored. Some psycho-biologists believe that emotion is not definable.

Despite this impression emotion may be thought of as any "feeling" state that exists beyond simple awareness regardless of whether the sensations are generated from within (via imagination) or from without (via environment). Emotion must be awakened through visual, olfactory, auditory, taste, or tactile perception, understanding or imagination. Perception, in a broad sense, is reached whenever external input becomes usable information.

Debate exists as to whether perception may produce awareness completely divorced from emotion. This is theoretically possible. An example of perception that probably does not evoke emotion is our vague awareness of the threshold we cross as we pass through a door. Much of what we see in peripheral vision is perception that is a semi-conscious awareness, devoid of any emotion—devoid of any pleasure—displeasure component. This type of perception may be considered a pure cortical function independent of any tie to the limbic system.

In all probability, emotion, regardless of whether it is a basic feeling state or is highly modified through learning, is never neutral. It probably always lies somewhere along a continuum of feelings from extreme pleasure of some form to extreme displeasure.

Pleasure may be considered to encompass any feeling that is desirable to the individual even if the gratification is derived from exposure to horror, pain, or tragedy. Such reactions, from sources that ordinarily and biologically produce unpleasant feelings, reflect the remarkable capacity of the neocortex to respond to the influences of acculturation that may modify, distort, or nullify innate predispositions and feeling patterns.

Pertinent Electro-Physiological Aspects

When a stimulating electrical current is passed into a pertinent area of the brain, actions may be produced directed toward defense of self, or aggressive patterns directed toward finding food. These behavior patterns, which are associated with preservation of the self, appear to be accompanied with facial and body expressions and movements suggestive of the unpleasant feelings of hunger, anger, anxiety, or fear. We may reasonably assume that these "feeling" states precede the actions as necessary precursors for the actions to take place.

Immediately adjoining the area of the brain associated with the production of self-preservation patterns is an area that appears to be related to species preservation. Stimulation of this area produces actions portraying sociability, such as grooming, courtship, and sexual activities. Experimental animals with electrode implants in this area of the brain will deliberately and repeatedly push the proper electrical switch to stimulate this region. Stimulation of this area in the squirrel monkey may even produce adduction of the thighs and penile erection while under anesthesia.[7] This suggests, though does not prove, the production of a desirable feeling state. M. Bishop, S. Elder, and Robert Heath, in their discussion of focal electrical stimulation data, commented that "…stimulation of activating and 'pleasure-inducing' regions has particularly benefited retarded, anhedonic, chronic schizophrenic patients."[8]

We may reasonably assume that feelings under the umbrella of pleasure are part of this pattern, but it is not as easy to recognize states of pleasure in lower mammals as it is to recognize rage or fear. This also holds true in some human beings. But because pleasure is not easily recognized in lower mammals does not mean it does not exist.

Some of the pathways flowing from the areas of the brain subserving self-preservation and species-preservation are quite close to each other. Electrical stimulation along this merging pathway can produce behavior patterns and physical changes such as actions of aggression with the appearance of fear and anger to be followed within a few seconds by penile erection.[9] This remarkable relationship suggests the presence of a spillover phenomenon that may be significant in our understanding of art. This spillover concept, probably made possible by the remarkably close anatomic relationship between the areas of self- and species-preservation, may well be the anatomic basis that helps explain how emotions of fear and pleasure are enabled to co-exist at the most basic level, and how pleasure may be derived from fear and pain. This concept suggests that there may be a lateral flow of impulses, via association fiber-tracts, that join the neural pathways subserving the forms of displeasure to the neural pathways subserving those of pleasure.

As a result of the growth of our tremendous new cortex, human beings are now able to markedly influence the primitive brain lying within the center of the human brain. As learning impacts upon this ability, we develop psychological processes of bewildering complexities.

In addition to the remarkable anatomy that, to some extent, may underlie the capability to derive pleasure from pain, another intriguing relationship apparently exists between our massive new cortex and the primitive brain that subserves emotion.

In the neuroscience studies of Birger Kaada is the suggestion that impulses generated within the cortex apparently find their way down to the limbic system quite easily, but impulses that originate within the limbic system do not as readily spread out to the cortex. They tend to remain relatively confined within this primitive brain.[10]

If this anatomical configuration is valid, it suggests that it may be relatively easy for information from the cortex to flow into the limbic system to influence feelings, and that learning, which is primarily a cortical function, can readily and markedly affect basic feelings. The unequal transfer of impulses between the cortex and the limbic system also suggests that feeling-state impulses circulating within the primitive brain are not as readily transmitted to the cortex. This anatomic quirk may partially explain the behavior of people who may be more prone to act impulsively without the full benefit of judgment resting in the cortex. It might also help to explain the strange conflict between what we feel and what we know. This remarkable neurological mechanism may predispose people to retain that treasured dichotomy of the human mind that allows us to more readily accept the conflict between what we may emotionally believe and what we understand. It also may account for the uncontrollable rage and temper that ignores the reason waiting to be used in the massive neocortex. The surge of emotion from the limbic system may throw the caution of the cortex to the winds. The individual prone to sudden rage may be so anatomically wired that the relative inability of impulses to flow from the limbic system to the cortex is more pronounced.

Since we have inherited the primitive brain, we may assume that our basic emotional and personality matrix reflects primitive patterns and feelings and therefore is primarily directed to seek and extend opportunities for feelings of pleasure and opportunities to avoid harm. Our overt emotional and behavior pattern may appear quite different as a result of our ability to learn and thereby affect the basic design. The human brain is a psycho-neurologic complex that functions as a unit. Our personality and behavior patterns reflect the total brain rather than simply primitive patterns.

Our highly developed cortex, so receptive to learning, not only permits intellectual growth, but also permits, though does not assure, control over the primitive reactions and feelings. Our cortex fosters the ability to respond to more subtle nuances. It hopefully enhances the ability to "feel" with greater intensity than can lower mammals. This potential of control enables the human being to repress as well as amplify basic feeling-states. As a result, the spectrum of human emotion extends far beyond primitive animalistic feelings. We have developed complex forms of love and compassion, anger and hate, arrogance, resentment, remorse, sadness, and lust for power.

The amazing degree to which human beings' basic emotional patterns may be altered by learning is most apparent when the forces for self-preservation, the most fundamental and most easily aroused biological behavior mechanisms, are negated. Many people willingly die for the protection of others or give up life for an abstract principle. The strong tie between basic feeling-states of fear and anxiety and their primal purpose to preserve life may become so attenuated that at times life is endangered. We even risk life to seek the tension, fear, and excitement of danger, despite the fact that the most primal force in nature is to preserve life. This paradox is especially, if not only, true in the human animal. Human beings seem to be the only mammals that deliberately endanger life for a form of pleasure. In regard to species-preservation, celibacy may be accepted with religious fervor with concealment or repression of sexuality.

The grand design of primal biochemical forces and of natural selection factors does not mean achievement of perfect design.

The massive neocortex of human beings may be considered an anatomic reflection of our enlarged intellectual potential, while the high ratio of the cortical neuronal population to that of the limbic system may be considered an anatomic reflection of our increased potential to amplify and control the emotional substrate. This control is especially noted in the influence exerted by the frontal lobe of the neo-cortex upon the limbic system as suggested by Walle Nauta. He states:

> it would seem justified to view the frontal cortex as the major—although not the only—neocortical representative of the limbic system. The reciprocity in an anatomical relationship suggests that the frontal cortex both monitors and modulates limbic mechanisms.[11]

Chapter Two

Basic Psychological Mechanisms

The following discussion identifies and explores the basic psychological mechanisms that underlie self-preservation and species-preservation and that serve as the substrate for the various forms of future pleasures. It is not directed toward the effect that life experiences or acculturation have upon these mechanisms. I am not in any way discussing the complex psychology of the mature human being, but only the foundation upon which the convolutions of meandering thoughts and emotions rest.

The following six psychological entities appear to be the basic mechanisms related to the achievement of pleasures.

1. Sexuality
2. Curiosity
3. Proprioception of pleasure
4. Release from displeasure (fear, pain, anguish)
5. Derivation from displeasure (fear, pain, anguish)
6. Mastery

Sexuality

Probably the most direct mechanism to achieve pleasure is through direct physical excitation of sexual feelings. The infant and child's penile erection noted during play is probably associated with pleasure that becomes, with repetition, more familiar to the infant who can then arouse that feeling with more purposeful genital play. This is probably the first learning that amplifies the pleasure associated with sexual overtones. Later, the thought of sex becomes pleasurable and serves as an impetus to sexual activity itself.

Curiosity

A second basic mechanism of direct excitement of pleasure, but not primarily sexual in character, is the remarkable phenomenon of curiosity. Curiosity, which exists in all vertebrates, is an inherited behavior pattern that serves multiple functions.

In all probability the underlying thrust of the puppy and human baby to explore crevices and corners in their surroundings is to seek adequate amounts of sensory stimulation. Studies of sensory deprivation reveal that low amounts of stimulation may result in inadequate development of the nervous system. Austin Riesen refers to this data. He states:

> the effect of early and prolonged sensory deprivation is to interfere with neural growth and function. Conversely, the use of sensory neurons results in the development to larger size, more complex structure, and increased physiological and behavioral reactivity....The striking evidence for a behavioral drive for light stimulation in monkeys...is a clear demonstration of a basic motivational component in stimulus-seeking behavior. Exploratory behavior appears to be no less physiologically motivated than are other drives that function to reduce need states.[1]

In essence curiosity fosters optimum development of the brain. A strong sense of curiosity helps maximize the growth and development of the central nervous system. Some studies show that rats that receive large amounts of sensory input, and live under conditions where the need to adapt and learn is demanded, may develop a thicker cortex compared to rats living in a simple environment.[2] M. Rosenzweig and E. Bennett report that "sensory deprivation early in life created adaptational difficulties in later life."[3]

Since curiosity is an important factor needed to enhance optimum development of the nervous system, we may reasonably conclude that some form of low intensity pleasure is associated with curiosity to encourage the tendency to be curious.

Besides its value for neural development, curiosity more overtly functions as a life-support mechanism. It is crucial for the development of a behavior pattern that enhances the ability to find potential sources for food. Although curiosity may lead to incidents that are disastrous or painful, such as curiosity about fire followed by intense burning pain, the principal thrust, which is genetically fostered, is toward neural enrichment. Until the moment of pain, a subtle sense of pleasure is probably associated with the feeling of curiosity. As a result of maximizing brain development, curiosity also produces a superior animal and therefore enhances the potential for both self-preservation and species-preservation. This suggests that if degrees of curiosity could be measured in a large segment of the population, it may reveal that the level of curiosity within individuals may be directly proportional to their level of intelligence.

When we reach the level of human beings, the tie between gratification and curiosity becomes more obvious. The process of fulfilling curiosity, of sensing and exploring, in itself is a source of pleasure. The enjoyment gained through curiosity is enhanced through conditioning. What is interesting and intriguing is tied to curiosity and is enjoyable. Exposure to a complex clock mechanism, space ship or satellite reflects this type of pleasure. Curiosity, aside from reflecting eagerness to know, incites imagination. Joseph Addison (1672–1719) referred to this relationship:

> Everything that is new or unconscious raises a pleasure in the imagination, because it fills the soul with an agreeable surprise, gratifies its curiosity, and gives it an idea of which it was not before possessed.[4]

But the pleasure derived from what is interesting appears to be at a lower level of emotional intensity than that derived from sensual pleasure.

Aristotle indirectly referred to the curiosity-pleasure concept when he suggested that "to learn gives the liveliest of pleasures" since the primary impetus to learning, aside from the desire to achieve, is curiosity.[5]

Curiosity as a source of pleasure is a factor in the joy of children at play in anticipation of what comes next. During play the pleasure of curiosity joins the pleasure associated with the kinesthetics of play with its increase in muscle tonus.

Proprioception and Pleasure

The awareness of body position, of the prideful stance, of muscle tonus, of conscious facial contortions has strong ties to emotion. Charles Darwin made the point that our facial expressions reflecting emotion are strongly related to our evolutionary pattern and therefore related to the facial expressions of other mammals. This concept has been supported by later studies. Although there are variations in the significance of the smile, one aspect of the smile is the feeling of comfort. The responding smile of a newborn child may be assumed to be associated with a feeling of contentment-pleasure almost certainly devoid of sexual overtones. This smile-pleasure relationship continues throughout life. As a result, the simple placement of facial features in a smile position through *mimicry* may be productive of a pleasant sense. If you are depressed and you place your facial features into a smile position you may begin to feel the pleasant reaction that is associated with and leads to smiling. This well-known phenomenon has recently been studied by Paul Ekman.[6]

Despite extreme cultural diversity throughout the world, the smile pattern is universally associated with the sense of security, contentment, comfort-pleasure. The explorer in the remote regions of Irian Jaya feels safe when greeted with a smile by a native warrior.

The proprioceptive aspect of energetic play in children, the three-year-old child's tendency to walk on its toes, the sense of well-being when standing very erect, all reflect the heightened physical tonus and stretch sensation associated with pleasure. This is probably a major factor in the enjoyment of the physical activity of sports.

Relief from Displeasure

A fourth mechanism concerns the type of pleasure associated with relief from displeasure. George Klein suggests that "the relief is itself experienced positively as pleasant."[7] R. Holt believes that the means by which the tension gets reduced is the source of the pleasure rather than the relief itself.

Several factors are involved. The sense of pleasure associated with the relief from displeasure may be an illusion of pleasure, as a feeling immediately juxtaposed to displeasure, a "pleasure" feeling that mimics, through comparative evaluation, the effect of pleasure. This is a negative aspect. The relief of intense pain belongs to this category of pleasure. "It feels so good when it stops hurting!" This kind of pleasure requires an immediate conscious awareness of unpleasantness. But if this negative aspect were the only factor, pleasure would probably not be pronounced.

At least three positive conditioning factors help associate this comfort type of pleasure with the relief from displeasure. They begin immediately after birth and convert what would have been only an illusion into a reality.

The three factors develop during the time a nursing infant is cradled in its mother's arms. One result of this close holding of the nursing child is the development of a sense of security synchronous with nullification of the anxiety associated with physical insecurity as well as the distress of hunger. This need for a sense of security was poignantly portrayed in Harry Harlow's photograph of a baby monkey holding on to a warm terry-cloth surrogate mother.[8]

It reflects the need of the infant to be held securely. The importance of holding the newborn infant securely may be best appreciated when viewing the grasping reflex and the Moro reflex of the child which is associated with the fear of falling. These movements reflect the genetic thrust of the infant to hold on to its mother. The pleasant sense of security counters the anxiety of falling.

A second factor is the sensually-oriented aspect of fondling the infant during nursing. As the infant senses the relief from the distress of hunger it is aware of the pleasurable sensual aspect of being cuddled and stroked. The development of pleasure associated with sensuality during the relief from the displeasure of hunger helps to develop the production of pleasure from displeasure in later life.

A third positive factor is based upon the relatively close anatomic relationship between sexuality and olfaction that still persists in human beings. Olfaction is phylogenetically intimately associated with mating in the primitive brain. Although there has been a significant evolutionary shift in human beings from the olfaction-sexuality relationship to a vision-sexuality relationship, olfaction still plays an important role in human beings. Taste, which is primarily dependent upon the sense of smell, and the mouth become closely allied to sex. The smell and taste of the mother become tied to the strong primitive pathways connecting smell to sex with its pleasurable aspects, a pleasure that occurs during relief from the distress of hunger.

These three factors help to establish the tie between the production of pleasure during relief from displeasure. The ability to derive pleasure as the distress of hunger is relieved reflects the ability to intertwine the feelings associated with self-preservation (hunger) with feelings normally associated with species-preservation. But despite these developmental aspects, most of the feelings of comfort-pleasure achieved as a release from displeasure reflect a sense of comfort when compared to the immediate memory of the preceding discomfort.

As a byproduct of these factors the sucking and mouthing patterns that are originally associated with the discomfort of hunger, which subserves self-preservation and is primarily non-sensual in character, reinforces the biological tie between oral mechanisms and sexuality discussed by Paul MacLean. He states:

> by stimulating parts of the amygdala one may obtain chewing and salivation, with partial erection....In other words, excitation in a region involved in oral mechanisms readily spills over into others concerned with genital function. This close neural relationship helps in understanding the intimate interplay of behavior in the oral and sexual spheres.[9]

The conditioning aspect combined with the biological factors may be the foundation underlying the pleasure of kissing, while the onset of comfort as hunger is relieved begins the process toward the enjoyment of food and the future gourmet's delight. With time and greater conditioning, what began only as a sense of comfort expands to a higher level of pleasure when hunger is satisfied and tastes are developed. With the development of food tastes, the pleasure associated with curiosity enters the picture and leads us to food experimentation, the gourmet's palate and the aesthetics of food.

Pleasure Derived Directly from Displeasure

The fifth mechanism related to the achievement of pleasure involves the development of pleasure directly from displeasure. The underlying factor that allows this close tie between opposite segments of the emotional spectrum is probably the anatomic configuration of the brain, although acculturation plays a significant role. The remarkably close juxtaposition of the areas of the brain related to self-preservation and species-preservation may allow the feeling states of displeasure to spill over into the area subserving pleasure.

This may be seen in the laboratory. When the area of the brain related to self-preservation is electrically stimulated, the impulses not only produce the expected unpleasant feelings and actions, but the impulses also spill over into the adjacent area concerned with species-preservation. This does not appear simply a question of the application of excess current or the leakage of current. Clinically, this spill-over effect may be seen when a male infant is frightened or angered at which time penile erection may occur. This is not to suggest that the infant is aware of pleasure, but we can reasonably assume that as the brain develops, the pleasure associated with penile erection becomes more acutely sensed. The neural pathways underlying this spill-over effect, after conditioning through learning, may become well-developed channels of communication that not only tie these two segments of the primitive brain more closely together, but also enhance the relationship between the massive neocortex and the limbic system. These relationships suggest an important anatomic neural mechanism that permits stimuli felt primarily as displeasure to produce a sense of pleasure.

The potential to gain pleasure from displeasure has significant implications. It is theoretically conceivable that people can learn to obtain pleasure from almost any type of input including intense pain. The tremendous influence of learning upon these pathways permits the development of gratification to be obtained from danger, fear, deprivation, anger, tragedy, and anguish. This conditioning partially accounts for the gratification obtained by the pyromaniac's fear-inducing fire, the masochist's pleasure through utilization of pain and fear of pain, and the sadist's gratification gained through expression of aggression. This close tie between pleasure and displeasure gives biologic support to Freud's statement that:

> The sexually-exciting influence of some painful effects such as fear, shuddering, and horror is felt by a great many people throughout life and readily explains why so many seek opportunities to experience such sensations.[10]

He also stated that:

> A number of persons report that they experienced the first signs of excitement in their genitals during fighting or wrestling with playmates....The infantile connection between fighting and sexual excitement acts in many persons as a determinant for the future preferred course of their sexual impulse.[11]

At levels in the evolutionary tree below that of human beings, it appears doubtful that any animal deliberately exposes itself to elements of danger or displeasure except in defense of self, territory, or progeny. No known organism, except possibly primates, seeks out what is primarily unpleasant in order to obtain pleasure. This may seem doubtful to some scholars in view of patterns that appear venturesome in the lower animal. But such patterns are probably only manifestations of curiosity directed toward satisfying self and species-preservation needs as well as its thrust toward neural enrichment.

As a result of our tremendous learning capability, superimposed upon the anatomic spillover effect, the potential of fear and tension to serve as major sources of pleasure constitutes a major difference between human beings and lower mammals.

Mastery

The sixth psychological mechanism seems to apply in some degree to all basic psychological mechanisms. Mastery speaks of the desire and ability to reach a specific goal, to have control. The biological advantage of achieving mastery is that through the process of natural selection it enhances the creation of a stronger or more adaptive organism better apt to survive.

Mastery is phylogenetically related to self-preservation. This relationship is observed when the more dominant animal takes first opportunity to satisfy hunger. Mastery is also related to species-preservation as noted in the pattern of sexual battles between males during competition for a mate, as well as male aggression toward the female mammal to overcome hesitance of the sexual partner. Mastery, like curiosity, serves both self-preservation and species-preservation.

Associated with the activities involving mastery in the competition for food and mate, as with the phenomenon of curiosity, a feeling of pleasure slowly evolved to encourage the formation of masterful behavior. The pleasure of mastery feeds upon the pleasure of mastery.

Examples of mastery in the more primitive animal include the pecking orders of chickens and the penile display actions of the squirrel monkey (Saimiri sciureus).[12] D.W. Ploog and Paul MacLean observed that even immature squirrel monkeys will display.[13]

Remnants of genital communication exist today among certain tribes in the use of wooden house guards and stone territorial markers with erect phallus, as well as in the child's tendency to display his or her genitals. MacLean suggests that covering the sexual organs is a behavior pattern designed to reduce the social tensions arising from archaic aggressive impulses to display. This could be a factor in the development of modesty.[14]

The phenomena of mastery and the pleasure associated with it accounts, to some degree, for the pleasure obtained from the control of fear; the negation of insecurity; the establishment of order out of disorder; the recognition of what was difficult to recognize, the sudden insight to the core of a dilemma; the solving of a complex problem; the concept of victory; climbing mountains; the achievement of power; the accumulation of wealth; the control over personal inadequacies; the experience of the child who has successfully tied its shoes for the first time; and, as our behavior patterns become complex, even altruism and philanthropy with its unconscious feeling of mastery over people and events.[15]

The erect stance of human pride, as a reflection of mastery, is related to the strut and body tightness of the stud who wins his territory and his mare. Mastery arouses pleasure that is probably more closely akin to the type of pleasure surrounding sexuality than to the pleasure derived from curiosity. During the achievement of mastery, elements of anxiety and tension exist. This close tie between tension and sensuality may, with learning, become enmeshed and expanded to the degree that some may seek most of their sexual satisfaction through stress and conflict.

Mastery is a significant element in enhancing the preceding five sources of pleasure. As we continue the process of gaining pleasure, regardless of which basic modality is brought into play, we not only gain what is expected but also gain an added dimension of pleasure through the mastery of achieving it. This is especially true when the behavior is consciously directed toward satisfying our desires.

There is therefore at least a two-fold basis for the development of pleasure under most circumstances: (1) the primary source and (2) the pleasure through mastery of gaining it. The mere recall of mastery may become exciting. The day-dream leading to the Walter Mitty syndrome reflects the pleasure of mastery. The sensation associated with the awareness of a strong ego is pleasurable.

Regardless of how we may modify or control the primitive brain with our massive cortex, the emotional substance of human beings remains a reflection of the primitive emotive stance. Regardless of how deeply they are hidden in the unconscious, we probably should assume that the primitive emotional patterns or feeling states underlie all human emotions. The development of complex variations of emotional overtones, whether it be the taste of fine wine, the pleasure of music, enjoyment of tragic opera, or watching the sun filter through deep woodlands, reflects the ability of the human mind to reach ineffable areas of awesome spirituality, but that does not imply that totally different basic mechanisms are operating. Those magnificent moments are still based upon primal feelings associated with sensuosity, curiosity, fear, and mastery. Our basic animalistic feelings may be hidden, but not destroyed.

Bowlby strongly supports this position:

> Those who dispute the view that there is in man behavior homologous with what in other species is traditionally called instinctive, have a heavy onus of proof on their hands. In respect of man's anatomical and physiological equipment a continuity in structure with that of other species is unquestionable. In respect of his behavioral equipment continuity of structure may be less evident, but were continuity to be totally absent all we know of man's evolution would be contradicted. What is far more probable than absence of continuity is, therefore, that the basic structure of man's behavioral equipment resembles that of infra-human species but has in the course of evolution undergone special modifications that permit the same ends to be reached by a much greater diversity of means. The early form is not superseded; it is modified, elaborated, and augmented but it still determines the overall pattern.[16]

Chapter Three

Emotion and Its Relationship to the Arts

Before trying to relate basic emotional mechanisms to the arts, I would like to refer to Sigmund Freud's reference to music. He said:

> ...works of art do exercise a powerful effect on me,...this has occasioned me...to explain to myself what their effect is due to. Whenever I cannot do this, as for instance with music, I am almost incapable of obtaining any pleasure. Some turn of mind in me rebels against being moved by a thing without knowing why I am affected and what it is that affects me.[1]

This statement by the father of psychoanalysis is intimidating. In the face of Freud's reluctance to explain this phenomenon, it is with trepidation that I discuss possible modalities that suggest how music as well as the other arts affect us at the most basic level, but not why one form or level of art is more exciting than another.

The Formative Period

During the formative period of infancy and early childhood almost all incidents are associated with nuances of emotion. The type, quality, and pattern of sounds heard during moments of comfort and pleasure become entwined, while the quality of sounds associated with startle, fright and sometimes pain become equally entwined. These relationships, through the process of conditioning, serve as the basis for future reactions to similar sound patterns, regardless of whether they are musical or random sounds.

Such conditioning is not limited to sound. During this period of life, all sensations (auditory, olfactory, visual, proprioceptive, tactile, and taste) become linked to the emotions evoked at the time of exposure to these sensations. The sensuous and calming feeling evoked by a delicate caress may subsequently be evoked by imagination of such actions.

Aside from this direct linkage, since all sensations are potentially anatomically related to each other through the development of new neural pathways, the emotional patterns associated with any one sensory modality become closely intertwined with other sensory modalities in the developing mind of the young child. The emotions associated with touch become tied to those of vision, etc.

The effect of conditioning in the relationships productive of the various forms of pleasure, when combined with the pleasures derived from curiosity and mastery, serve as part of the substructure upon which the enjoyment of all the arts stand. This holds true despite the distance between complex music and the sound patterns or movements of childhood. This tie, in its simplest form, accounts for the feelings of tenderness, softness, and warmth felt with a lullaby: a return of feelings experienced with the soothing sounds of cuddling, stroking, and nursing.

As emotions become more complex as a result of learning, the original close tie between primary feeling states and specific events, sounds, or movements fades to remain hidden in memory. Although the arts may penetrate and arouse unconscious feelings, rarely are incidents recalled that were associated with those sensations early in life.

The distance between feelings associated with early sound patterns and the emotions evoked by Beethoven is immense. This distance reflects the complexity of the psychodynamic convolutions, but despite the complexity of such emotional development, the reaction has been built upon patterns set down early in life that in turn are intimately tied to primitive animalistic emotions.

There is a genetically driven pattern that apparently predisposes toward the feeling of alarm and fear upon exposure to sudden unexpected loud sound or movement. This is reflected in the startle reaction (Moro reflex) of the newborn to sudden movements or loud sounds. On the other hand, quiet rhythmic sounds and gentle movement are associated with feelings of calm. These relationships establish the basic patterns that later are modified through learning. They are applicable to all art forms, but especially to dance and music. Except for the factors of rhythm and unexpected sudden loud sounds, the emotional reaction associated with music is a function of conditioning. This suggests that any type of music may become a future source of pleasure, especially if heard during moments of pleasure or release from displeasure during the formative years of life. In this regard it is of interest to note that infants portray discomfort when exposed to dissonance.[2]

The flowing caress of a parent's loving hand associated with the smooth flow of gentle sound or the sudden impulse of movement associated with tension, force, and pain become meaningful combinations. The dynamic relationships between a body stance and its feel or between a movement and its sensation become entwined and unconsciously recalled during similar relationships in the future. Aside from the effect of learning, the direction or patterns of movement and subsequent feelings also appear to be tied to normal physiology, similar to the feeling of a smile produced by the deliberate positioning of facial musculature into a smile. This accounts for the smile as a universal symbol that crosses all cultural lines.

The flow of upward or downward directions in sound or body movements appears to have a specific relationship to emotional patterns. It is natural during periods of intense fatigue or depression for the human body to show a downward sag of muscle and loss of body tonus associated with a feeling of heaviness. The fallen shoulders, the limp hand, and the downward curve of the mouth are commonly associated with sadness, depression, and fatigue. These patterns are commonly seen in primates. A relationship exists between these movements and positions with downward vectors and the feeling states and images associated with them. These are not learned but genetically imposed patterns that become intensified with learning.

If we extrapolate these relationships, a descending sequence in a musical theme, a line hanging limply in painting, and a downward sag of the shoulders in dance, are likely to produce feelings of quietness, sadness, or fatigue. But this does not mean that music or line in a descending pattern cannot give rise to soaring and ecstatic moments of emotion, nor that music or line in an ascending sequence cannot give rise to feelings of mystery and sadness. We must appreciate the tremendous distance between the pattern of primal biological relationships, unaltered by acculturation, and the effect of acculturation upon those patterns. Nevertheless, the general characteristics of the downward line or descending scale is usually more conducive to some aspect of melancholy, sadness, sense of quietness, or sense of fatigue. At least it is easier to evoke such feelings with downward vectors. This will be discussed in more detail later. On the same basis, increased tonus associated with the upward movement of the body is more likely to evoke feelings of elan, excitement, and happiness. People who are on a consistent exercise program with increased strength and body tonus are known to have a better sense of well-being; an increased sense of vitality. The physiological relationship between the pleasant feeling associated with increased strength and body tone is not such a distant cousin to the pleasure associated with the surging tightness of sexual activity.

It is within this context that the composer and choreographer, through their music and dance, intuitively incite and manipulate the emotions of their audience. When this is augmented by inciting the imagination through curiosity, the emotional impact, the pleasure, and the aesthetic significance of the work increases.

Rhythm

Another inherited factor and possibly the most important factor in the enjoyment of the arts, especially music and dance, is rhythm. Rhythmicity is deeply ingrained in all living tissue. There is an inherent biologic rhythm in all forms of life, and broad geophysical rhythms that affect life.

The rhythmic beat of the heart and the rhythmic arhythmia associated with respiration are obvious reflections of the rhythm in all living tissue. The circadian rhythm of sleep and wakefulness, of night and day, as well as the thirteen and seventeen-year cyclic lifespan of the cicada are reflections of broader rhythmic patterns. The moon changes and we have months, and within the months women have the rhythmic pattern of menses. There are bio-geophysical rhythms of exquisite precision. Each year between April and June a swarming occurs of the grunion, a small fish, upon the beaches of California a few minutes after the exact time of the month when the sun and the moon are cooperating to produce the highest tide of the month.[3]

Rhythm is everywhere and in every living thing. It is difficult to move arhythmically. The regularity of rhythm, or its regular irregularity forces a sense of order into the dance. It is as difficult to jump arhythmically as it is difficult to breath arhythmically. The primitive repetitive jump becomes a dance, its rhythmicity a natural physiological attribute. With rhythm as its base, evolutionary forces probably played a role in the development of music and dance, and possibly the visual arts as well. During tribal rites and excitement the primitive beings, the precursors of Homo sapiens, with superior talent in rhythm, may, via the process of natural selection, select a mate with similar attributes leading to a slight shift of the bell curve of rhythm to the right. Although not directed toward self or species preservation, such an adaptive process certainly enhances the quality of life. Sounds that are repeatedly expressed lead into rhythmic chant because of greater ease physiologically, and that leads to song. Rhythm disciplines chaotic sound and movement. The rhythmic movement of the conductor's baton is not the rhythm itself, it only reflects the rhythm sensed within the conductor. Rhythm is a recognizable pattern of time.

There are at least two types of rhythm. First is the rhythm that is evenly paced with only minor variations. It is this type of rhythm that the developing fetal brain must first sense: the mother's heartbeat and the gentle rhythmic sway of her respiration, a repetitive, relatively even pulsation, probably soothing, calming and comforting in effect. Then there is the paced rhythm of increasing tempo and force reaching the peak of excitement in sexuality.

Max Schoen suggests, "Marked rhythm as an element in music is the chief factor in arousing the feeling of happiness and the feeling of excitement or stir."[4] Since the most dynamic, most pleasurable phenomenon per unit time in the human being and possibly all mammals is the crescending explosive rhythm of orgasm, it is possible that within the subtle, and oftentimes not so subtle, incitement of this most conscious of rhythmic acts lies part of the pleasure derived from music and dance.

An enhancement to the impact of rhythm is the presence of some degree of arhythmia, irregularity, or as Carl Seashore describes it, "grouping."[5]

Rhythm is vital to the existence of dance, music, and poetry, but it alone does not make music or any art form. The enjoyment of Johann Sebastian Bach or George Gershwin is based upon much more than a simple relationship between the musical beat and the rhythm of orgiastic pleasure or the comfort associated with the soothing rhythm of the heartbeat. But regardless of how subtle rhythm may be, part of our gratification from music and dance is related to its rhythmic flow and its tie to sensuality. As W. Bardas expressed it, "The joy of music must be rooted in pleasure feelings, which cannot originate in refined aesthetical satisfaction but only in most primitive, common, therefore to all mankind, instinctual gratification of drives."[6]

Only with persistent exposure and conditioning can a person enjoy music when the pulse is too vague to be readily sensed. This is a major hurdle that some contemporary composers face when they compose music with an exceedingly subtle or hidden rhythmic structure. In such situations, the primal factor of curiosity, interestedness, becomes quite pertinent in the production of pleasure. Interest as a source of pleasure is rarely if ever productive of pleasure as intense as that associated with distinct rhythm that relates the music more definitely to sensuosity. Interest as it applies to all art forms is the least powerful impetus to an aesthetic reaction. When someone looks at a painting or sculpture and states that it is interesting, that reflects the blandest reaction to art. That someone would display a urinal as sculpture may be of interest as an act but not interest as the beginning of an aesthetic reaction.

In regard to poetry, rhythm or cadence when joined by the rhyme of words enhances the intimacy with the thought and word. This intimacy awakens emotional overtones. Emotion becomes bound to ideas or words that are often devoid of any obvious emotional content. Through the enhancing effect of rhythm and sound, the mental or vocal feel of the word or the phrase that may be termed its weight, its color, or its look, new perceptions are born. We are then able to embark upon a word or thought association that enlarges thoughts and arouses feelings beyond what a given word would ordinarily suggest.

Poetry stirs up poignant memories, stirs imagination to feel what has not been felt, awakens understanding, entices us to feel the potential in human qualities surrounding us, and elevates our ability to sense the awesome that lies hidden in our lives.

Dylan Thomas stressed a different aspect of poetry and the significance of words when he wrote a letter to a student of poetry.

> I had fallen in love with words...the words alone. What the words stood for, symbolized, or meant, was of secondary importance; what mattered was the sound of them as I heard them...these words were, to me, as the notes of bells, the sounds of musical instruments, the noises of wind, sea and rain, the rattle of the milk carts, the clopping of hooves on cobbles, the fingering of branches on a window pane,...I did not care what the word said,...I cared for the shape made in my ears; I cared for the colours the word cast...on my eyes...I fell in love...at once, and am still at the mercy of words....[7]

Poetry is probably most appreciated when recited, when heard, at which time the cadence, the rhythm, is heard, and the music within the word is more readily sensed. The word is inert. Poetry is released in the imagery provoked by the word. This is amplified by the sound of the word. Memorization assumes importance. George Steiner comments, "To learn by heart is to afford the text or music an in-dwelling clarity and life force...[it] deepens our grasp of the work...."[8]

Since language is often inadequate to express emotional nuances, metaphor is commonly used to help bring insight into the understanding of feeling. Pinchas Noy referred to this problem: "Art's function to widen the scope of language and mold its means so that they may be utilized to express all human experience which ordinary language cannot convey is best demonstrated in poetry."[9]

Curiosity

The biological construct of curiosity leads us to explore the musician's approach to sound, the dancer's next movement and the poet's sensitivity and insights, whether it be about the mystery of bird migration, the sense of joy in rain, the mysticism of faith, or the nuance of a word. Curiosity reflects the perceiver's active participation in the art process. As interest develops, the factor of curiosity expands, and association patterns and their feeling states are aroused, resulting in intimacy and empathy with the work. Within the process of curiosity itself arises the primal pleasure of curiosity. As insight is gained, this element of pleasure is enhanced by an additional sense of gratification fostered by the mechanism of mastery that is brought into play with the onset of insight. This increased awareness sharpens and intensifies our focus. Within the intensity of this rapport exists the "atmosphere of infinite suggestion…" of Andrew C. Bradley,[10] a suggestion that permits extrapolation of that insight or rapport into all elements of life. Bradley suggests that, "The poet speaks…of one thing, but in this one thing there seems to lurk the secret of all…his meaning seems to beckon away beyond itself…."

This extrapolation potential may be more prominent in poetry than other art forms. It may be because of this potential that poetry is considered by many to be the "Queen of the Arts."

Curiosity, as it relates to music, is aroused by the unknown direction that the flow of sound and sculptured silence will take, the manner themes are developed, the character of the rhythm and its variations, and the sensing of nuances previously unrecognized. In this respect, the element of curiosity, and hence interest with resultant pleasure, is especially prominent in classical music where symphonic and chamber music appear to contain an endless supply of fresh nuances to be sensed.

Noy describes this seeking of nuances:

> The fourth movement of Mozart's Jupiter symphony…[is] built on five different themes….You can enjoy listening to…nothing more than the single melodic line and its rhythmical beats….But you may receive an even greater pleasure by following various ingenious combinations of two, three or four themes and the inversions from beginning to end…you will achieve greatest pleasure of all if you succeed to follow all five melodic lines of the symphony to their climax…where they converge into a magnificent five-part counterpointal structure.[11]

Content

Another factor to be considered in the development of pleasure in some of the arts is the absence of specified content. The lack of words, story line, or recognizable visual images allows us to be free of directed thoughts. We are not directed to think of a specific concept or image such as war, landscape, or horses. When we listen to a symphony, the mind is not forced to focus upon any given concept. The emotions are free to respond within the framework of the individual's experience and sensitivity.

We need not be aware of the artist, his or her motivation, thoughts, or intent in order to respond to the work. We need only permit the flow of sound, line, or movement with its variations in quality and rhythm to impinge upon the mind. Whatever preconceived concept exists is what the perceiver alone may wish to construct upon the artist's work. It is true that the musical form may suggest an image that the composer wishes to convey, an image that the perceiver may or may not perceive. To listen to Vivaldi's "Four Seasons" without knowledge of its title and the composer's intent would probably not elicit the feelings associated with images of the seasons.

This freedom allows us to participate with music or nonobjective visual art with an unrestrained and uninhibited flow of imagination and feelings. We are permitted a unique opportunity to feel unfettered, to flow with time, to emotionally fly free of detailed thought-processes, free to enter into an amorphous feeling state.

Regardless of whether the emotion is more obviously sensual as with the music of the tango, or more subtle as in a Mozart quartet, regardless of whether the effect is more delicate or more pulsating, realistic images are usually not evoked. If the listener is totally involved, conceptualization of images is probably absent. By this I mean conceptualization tied to the music, not of daily problems and decisions using the music, or the time during which the music is being played, as a background element. This is not music involvement; this is music escape. A large percentage of listeners and viewers are not capable of letting go, of allowing their minds to freely follow the emotional flow. Many people become only partially involved when exposed to any of the arts, especially music. The ability to obtain full measure of enjoyment from music is dependent upon the ability to become immersed in it. This necessitates or is accompanied by, as Charles S. Myers expressed it, a "self forgetfulness"[12] that is difficult to achieve.

The significance of the absence of conceptualization has been stressed by C.V. Ramana, who believed that one of the great advantages of music is that it penetrates the human consciousness rapidly without interfering concepts.[13]

The non-objective aspect of music permits two major psychological patterns to come into play. Firstly is the pleasure of relative tranquility as a result of freedom from thought. Unpleasant thoughts, our preoccupations and tensions of daily life are forgotten. There is a biological necessity for this physical and mental tranquility as reflected in the need for sleep. The release from prior tensions is probably a significant factor in the overall pleasurable effect of music aside from the positive factors gained by the full involvement with it. Max Schoen referred to this freedom when he said, "...music is in itself most abstract...and is least liable to suggest anything beyond itself, or in other words, it most easily induces the condition of mental detachment."[14]

Secondly, the new-found freedom may result in an unconscious cutting across the bonds of repressed feelings and thoughts, and thereby establish an opportunity for those restrained emotions to surface. Although emotions evoked through the arts are awakened in the unconscious as well as in the conscious, rarely, if ever, are feelings consciously related to early childhood relationships. Those early relationships remain hidden, but not lost in memory.

Sadness and Minor Mode Music

There are many musicologists who believe that music written in the minor mode is more prone to elicit feelings of sadness than music written in the major mode. Peter Kivy commented upon this relationship and mentioned:

> ...the wonderful moment in the finale of the Ninth Symphony when...Beethoven tinges the theme with grief by giving it a minor harmonization (in measures 205–206)....Why should the change merely of one note in a melody of itself change the whole character from joy to sorrow?...We must take a new look at musical expressiveness to find what it is that thus far has evaded us.[15]

George Steiner asks,"...why should G minor be the key of sadness?"[16]

W.J. Dowling and Dane Harwood, in their evaluation of the experimental studies of both K. Hevner and Scherer and Oshinsky, tend to confirm the general consensus.[17] M.P. Kastner and R.G. Crowder support this position and state:

> One of the compelling expressive devices in tonal music is the use of modes to suggest emotion: For most Western listeners, the minor mode suggests a negative emotional tone while the major mode has a more positive connotation, other things being equal.[18]

Numerous attempts to explain this impression have been made.

Hermann von Helmholtz discussed this issue. He assumed that the difference between the effects of the major and minor modes was tied to their different acoustic and spectral characteristics. He commented:

> The...element...introduced into the minor chord...is enough to give a mysterious, obscure effect to the musical character and meaning of these chords, an effect for which the hearer is unable to account...minor chords are especially adapted to express mysterious obscurity.[19]

Deryck Cooke suggests that "the minor triad...being lower than the major third...has a "depressed sound."[20]

> To fall from the tonic to the dominant, taking in the mournful minor seventh and anguished minor sixth, is clearly to express an incoming painful emotion, an acceptance of, or yielding to grief...suffering; and the despair connected with death.[21]

On a slightly different tangent, the psychologist C.W. Valentine, following his experimental study of the effect of major and minor triads upon adults, suggested that:

> ...the general significance of the minor key for modern European ears is not due to an effect inherent in the relation of the notes in a minor interval, but is more probably the effect of association...with the custom of setting sad songs to minor keys....[22]

The psychologist Chester P. Heinlein also moved away from the assumption that there is a strong relationship between the semitone positions within the minor mode and the emotional spectrum. He suggested the most striking reason for the production of the two poles of the emotional spectrum was not so much the major or minor key aspect but the quality of the sound as to its loudness and pitch. Loud or high pitched chords were inclined to produce excitement while quiet and low pitched chords were inclined to produce calming or melancholic effects generally construed as being associated with the minor key. These reactions took place regardless whether the music was in the major or minor mode.[23]

Robert G. Crowder takes Heinlein to task and suggests that contrary to Heinlein's interpretation of his data, the proper conclusion is that the data gives "...overwhelming support for the conventional connotation..." and does not negate the general impression as to the impact of minor mode music.[24]

Despite the impression that minor mode music is more prone to elicit feelings of sadness, minor mode music is certainly capable of eliciting uplifting, joyous and majestic feelings while major mode music is very capable of producing intense feelings of pathos and sadness.

The basis for the effect of music upon our emotions is much more complex than the factor of a minor or a major mode construct. The context as to when and where the music is played, the time, the character, age and the historical background of the audience, the rhythm and especially the timbre of the music all play crucial roles as to whether the effect is one of elation, pensiveness, sadness or any feeling along the emotional spectrum.

But, aside from all other factors, there is something about minor mode music that has a unique relationship to the development of melancholy. What is it?

Johan Sundberg's study of speech characteristics and voice effects revealed that "Phonation frequency descends slowly with sorrow...and is almost falling monotonously toward the end of the phrase." He mentioned the work of Kotlyar and Morosov who in their study of the songs performed by eleven professional singers noticed that all acoustic parameters including tempo was slowest for songs reflecting sorrow.[25]

During the past forty years, I have been exposed to frequent tragedy during my work as a neurosurgeon. When informing families that their loved one has a malignant brain tumor that cannot be totally removed, or parents that their child will eventually be blind, there is almost always an outpouring of grief with a change in body stance and tonus as well as weeping. After years of such routine exposure, I became aware of the quality of the sound of the wail of honest grief and its remarkable closeness in "feel" to much of the music written in the minor mode with its downward flow. The wail of true grief is unlike the sounds of crying heard during frustration, anger, pain or for the sake of propriety. In grief there is an expressive sagging of the voice reminiscent of the "feel" of the descending flow in minor mode music.

This subjective, empirical impression of the downward motion of the wail was recorded and objectively diagrammed by Manfred Clynes and Nigel Nettheim as part of their discussion of continuous and discrete sound frequency contours during the sounds of grief. The following diagram is adapted from their work.[26]

This downward pattern of sound resembling the flow of sound of the wail was also noted by Margarita Mazo during her spectrographic studies of lamenting. She noted that the wail and lament, aside from the timbre quality of the voice, "...is characterized by general pitch instability: a gliding pitch contour, modal structures without fixed scales, extensive use of microtonal intervals that continuously vary in size, an overall changing pitch level" that is characterized by a swift rise at the onset and then a significant downward slide. "The melodic contour...in lament disregarding inhalations and final exhalations is generally perceived as a descent...."[27]

The tendency for music in the minor mode to produce quietness, sadness, or melancholy, all else being equal, is probably not explainable as a function of physics, nor acculturation, but rather the result of a close similarity between the "feel" of sound of the descending semitones or microtones often recognized in minor mode music, and the natural quality and flow of sound of the human voice as humans wail and weep during moments of grief, sadness, and melancholy.

It is the remarkable similarity between the downward flow of the sound of the human wail of grief and the downward thrust in major and especially noted in minor mode music that I believe to be at least partly responsible for the minor mode's effect upon human emotion. It is the downward slide that is significant independent of the position of the semitones. Exposure to the flow of

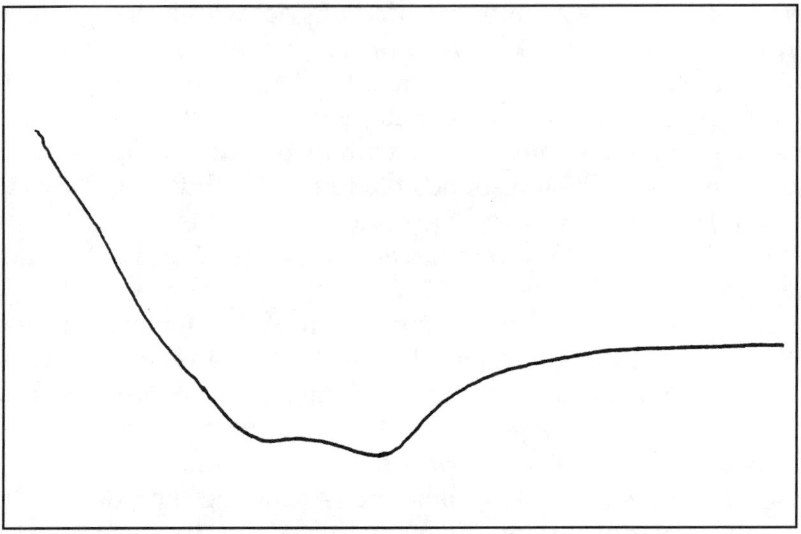

Figure 2: Contour of Wailing Sound During Expression of Grief
Adapted from *Music, Mind, and Brain: The Neuropsychology of Music*, ed. Manfred Clynes.

sound appears to evoke that relationship and touch those feelings. This characteristic of the human cry, in conjunction with Heinlein's explanation of the psychological significance of loudness and pitch, may be the crucial factors as to why minor mode music is more prone to produce sadness than music written in the major mode.

Since the pattern of the human wail is similar in all human beings despite cultural variations, the relationship between the human wail and music that resembles its downward flow may be a significant factor in the music of all cultures, aside from other factors that contribute to the effect of music. The saddening effect of such music may apply to those cultures whose musical idiom is characterized by microtones rather than specific intervals as the minor third or minor sixth which are Western cultural constructs.

Logical Sequence

The biological basis for the entity "logical sequence" is unclear. A strong sense of sequence is quite prominent among mathematicians and physicists as well as musicians. It may be remotely related to the strong rhythmic patterns that exist in all living matter, a pattern whereby the recognized sequence or rhythm is expected to continue. It is probably related to the need to avoid the insecurity and tension that is associated with incompleteness and indecision. When sequence has been established and continues to a logical or acceptable end, indecision and its anxiety fades. The unconscious fear of change, of the unknown next step is negated, and the comfort of order and of the familiar is maintained.

"Logical sequence" is an integral element in all the arts. It is the pattern of sequence of sound, silence, movement, phrase, or thought that resonates with the anticipatory sense of sequence within human beings. This sense is directed toward a feeling of continuity, an unconscious requirement for reasonable tie between successive entities, and a reasonable resolution of tension. It is crucial in the development of cohesiveness. Its use in the arts lies in the manipulation of the delay of resolution that permits the emotions to be more readily stressed until finally the tension is resolved and the character of its unity is exposed.

Logical sequence is most obviously sensed in the flow of music and dance. Who has not conducted a symphony with grand gestures while listening at home to music, or sensed the power of the composer by anticipating the direction of the next musical phrase? Logical sequence is quite significant in poetry and prose, and is important, but less obvious, in visual art.

The pattern of flow of what the eye sees as it moves between color masses and objects in painting is analogous to the sequence of sound and pause in music, form and space in painting and sculpture, and the completion of a body movement in dance. The positioning and sequence of space and silence is as important as the more obvious sequence of sound, color, or word. When all elements are tied together, a cohesive unit has been established, and unity or resolution has been achieved. Within the sense of completeness lies an element of safety and feeling of comfort through negation of indecision and insecurity.

The ability to sense the next sequence brings into play the mechanism of mastery. Gratification derived from the resultant incitement of mastery is significant although usually subtle. In the midst of enjoying music or dance, the perceiver, although participating in the sense of sequence, is usually not consciously aware of the details of the sequence but is immersed in the overall "feel."

Mastery

The pleasure derived from mastery is pervasive throughout all art forms. It is brought into play when the music elicits a feeling of majesty with its concomitant sense of power, or when stress and conflicts incited by the musical flow or story line are finally resolved and thereby mastered. Control over insecurity appears with the relief of musical tension, as when the prolonged note that seems to continue without end is finally terminated and the musical phrase resolved. The pleasure due to mastery enhances the primary pleasure derived from music or any of the art forms.

A pleasure through mastery that applies more specifically to classical music occurs when you suddenly become aware of the subtle nuances within the musical phrase following repeated listening to the music. This complements the pleasure derived from curiosity discussed in the example of Mozart's symphony. In general, classical music is more complex with more hidden nuances than popular, ballad, or folk music. The complexity demands that the listener be more focused upon and more knowledgeable about the musical phraseology in order to gain the full measure of pleasure from the music. In accomplishing this end mastery appears. This is supported by the studies of Margaret Washburn, *et al.*, who found that music which is more intricate, more difficult, and more challenging will result in a greater sense of pleasure as understanding is achieved.[28] This does not necessarily mean that we can equate greater complexity with greater degree of pleasure, only with greater interest in the search for more elements to be mastered. This suggests a lesser tendency toward boredom upon repeated exposure to the same musical score.

The sense of mastery that evolves during the flow of emotion usually remains unrecognized, lodged in the unconscious, while the pleasure produced is felt.

The factor of mastery, although prominent in the enjoyment of classical music is especially applicable to art forms with content such as the literature of drama. This can be most easily understood if we discuss tragedy, which is a remarkably common theme in much art.

Tragedy in the Arts

Intriguing questions arise. Why does such heavy outpouring of tragedy occur in the arts, especially literary art and opera? How can we enjoy it when tragedy is something we all wish to avoid and the feelings it engenders are basically unpleasant? Why do audiences speak of Verdi's Othello or Shakespeare's Hamlet as beautiful despite human suffering, sadness, anger, fear, anguish, apprehension, pathos and violent death?

Joseph Addison referred to this dilemma:

> ...how it comes to pass that such passions as are very unpleasant at all other times, are very agreeable when excited by proper descriptions...that we should take delight in being terrified or dejected by a description, when we find so much uneasiness in the fear or grief which we receive from any other occasion?[29]

The apparent close relationship between pleasure and displeasure is one of the most intriguing aspects of human emotion. Their frequent coexistence may be seen in the pleasure derived from tragedies in drama, opera, as well as in visual art. The thrill associated with exposure to danger reflects this same pleasure-displeasure relationship in social behavior.

Max Dessoir comments that "What is tragic in ordinary life is indeed sad, but not tragic in the artistic sense. Artistic tragedy has splendour and grandeur."[30]

In visual arts, the coexistence of pleasure and displeasure may be recognized and analyzed by a study of the painting "The Fifth of May" by Goya. This painting of tragic, fearful, and awesome moment arouses disturbing emotions. Through insight into tragedy poetically expressed, we gain a sense of nobility in the human spirit. Interest and curiosity is aroused which lead to gratification that lies hidden under the more obvious awe and regret at the horror of the situation. This may also be seen in a different manner by a study of the painting "Les Souliers" by Van Gogh. The sight of a stranger's dilapidated, odoriferous old shoes would not be expected to evoke pleasurable sensations, but in this painting the artist portrays old shoes so as to arouse poignant sensations. The viewer is no longer only aware of someone's old shoes, but is struck by a sense of forlornness, loneliness, and quiet anquish. The shoes become symbolic of a sadder aspect of life. Again pleasure via interest and curiosity is aroused, as well as the pleasure of mastery derived from an unconscious "awareness" of absence of that sadness from our lives.

Susanne K. Langer states, "Few people know why tragedy is a source of deep satisfaction...." Then she attempts to explain why it is so: "...the real source is the joy of revelation, the vision of a world wholly significant, of life spending itself and death the signature of its completion."[31] But this contortion still does not seem to explain why tragedy is a source of deep satisfaction.

Aristotle's reference to katharsis (catharsis) focuses on this "complex transformation of feelings."[32] Katharsis is a Greek word meaning to purge, to purify.[33] A vagueness to the term suggests a vicarious cleansing or washing away of distressful feelings associated with tragedy, possibly reducing the intensity of those feelings, or converting those feelings to compassion.

I know of no simple answer to these questions, but part of the answer may lie hidden within biology.

The most easily aroused emotions, namely apprehension and fear are related to self preservation. This appears true in experimental animals and in human beings. It is much easier to frighten lower mammals or human beings than to arouse their curiosity or sexuality. Any form of pleasure can almost always be overwhelmed and immediately negated by a sudden threat to life.

It is therefore probably easier, from a purely psychological point of view, for an artist to arouse his or her audience's emotion by suggesting apprehension and fear rather than tranquility. Is the frequency of tragedy in the arts the result of the artist coldly taking calculated advantage of this understanding, or does its frequency reflect what is most easily felt by the artist? It is also possible that the mediocre artist, in order to compensate for artistic inadequacy, will deliberately portray images associated with the tragic or frightening emotions of life in the hope that by the simple awakening of emotion the perceiver will accept the work as good art.

When we are in the ambience of artistic tragedy we may unconsciously detach ourselves from the vision of tragedy in order to understand its source, its potential ramifications, and the machinations underlying the scene of tragedy. In the process, we modify the initial shock associated with intense involvement with "reality" to involvement with detached reality. This is usually accomplished unconsciously, but at times when we appear to become overwhelmed with tension, we may achieve the same result through a conscious and deliberate "sitting back."

George Santayana suggests:

> since all moderate excitement is pleasant, there is nothing strange in the fact that the representation of evil should please; for the experience is evil by virtue of the pain it gives; but it gives pain only when felt with great intensity. Observed from afar, it is a pleasing impression; it is vivid enough to interest, but not acute enough to wound.[34]

At a more superficial level I do not doubt that some people may derive pleasure from the observation of tragedy on a sadistic basis as expressed in the German word "Schadenfreude," that refers to the malicious pleasure some people obtain from another person's misfortune.

It is difficult to identify which fundamental modality, each of which have been markedly elaborated upon by the input from living and learning, is being used to bring the many different forms of pleasure into play. In Schadenfreude, a major element is probably some form of mastery.

Let us approach this problem from a different direction. I suggest that the pleasure derived from tragedy as expressed through the arts is fundamentally related to three elements: 1. pleasure as a direct result of exposure to the excitement and tension of the dramatic process; 2. pleasure as a byproduct of fascination, an intense form of curiosity; and 3. pleasure as derived from mastery in the awareness that we are not actively involved in the tragic scene. But how do we permit these mechanisms to function in the face of tragedy?

In regard to the first element, pleasure via tension, we may recall the spillover concept discussed in Chapter One whereby stress, excitement, and tension may directly lead to sensual pleasure. This phenomenon is reflected in the penile erection of the infant when suddenly frightened. The crossover potential may be a subtle factor that aids the production of pleasure when exposed to horror movies or tragedy in plays.

Curiosity as another factor in the production of pleasure during exposure to tragedy in the arts was alluded to by Yrjo Hirn when he referred to the power of fascination.

> The more we can compel ourselves to contemplate with cool and clear attention the causes and manifestations of…high strung states, the more we are also able to master them…strong fear can be vanquished, if only we can succeed in diverting all our attention to its objective source and "stare the danger in the face." When the attention is concentrated and intensified to the utmost degree, it may even, as in the case of fascination, entirely prevent, to our own danger, the very rise of this self-preserving emotion. During the exposure to tragic art so irreconcilable…is the conflict between emotional excitement and intellectual activity, that the latter…must neutralize the excess of feeling.[35]

Inherent in Melvin Rader's perceptive phrase, "dynamic calmness" so apparent in the facial expression and body language of audiences in the presence of great tragic art, is the element of fascination with the dramatic process.[36] The curiosity of the audience is so intense that they are driven to continue to see what will happen, and how and why it will happen.

The third element relates to the possible development of pleasure secondary to tension. This holds true especially when fear is detached as it is in a play. Fear is felt, but sub-consciously we are aware that it is someone else's problem. With this subliminal awareness, the pleasure derived from mastery becomes part of the process. The mastery occurs in the sense that we are not truly in danger; therefore, we have mastery over the insecurity sensed in the drama. Addison refers to this phenomenon:

> …it does not arise so properly from the description of what is terrible, as from the reflection we make on ourselves at the time….When we look on such hideous objects, we are not a little pleased to think we are in no danger of them. We consider them at the same time, as dreadful and harmless; so that, the more frightful appearance they make, the greater is the pleasure we receive from our own safety….the misfortunes we read in history or poetry, either as past, or as fictitious…rises in us insensibly, and overbears the sorrow we conceive for the sufferings of the afflicted.[37]

I doubt Addison's concept that the degree of pleasure received through the unconscious sense of mastery is directly proportional to the degree of tragedy in the arts. The portrayal of more profound anguish does not translate itself into greater pleasure. Pleasure derived through mastery upon exposure to tragedy in painting or theater is extremely subtle. Pleasure is probably never consciously part of the process except in the very insensitive human being endowed with a twinge of cruelty reflecting Schadenfreude.

Although we may have a strong sense of participation when we are exposed to tragedy in art, we are not truly aware of the gratification felt during those moments. We are primarily aware of a sense of intense involvement and tension which is unpleasant.

Underlying this complex psychodynamic is a mechanism tied to mastery without which the gratification derived from tragic art may not be possible. It is an unconscious or semi-conscious detachment from reality; "I am not really involved." The ability to gain this perspective is in great part explained by Edward Bullough who considered the problem of involvement and described the concept of distance. This concept becomes especially important when tension is a significant factor. Distance is not simply distance in terms of space or time, but rather, "psychical distance." This is most accurately described by Edward Bullough himself:

> A short illustration will explain what is meant by "Psychical Distance." Imagine a fog at sea; for most people it is an experience of acute unpleasantness…it is apt to produce feelings of peculiar anxiety, fears of invisible dangers…warning calls soon tell upon the nerves of the passengers, and that…expectant, tacit anxiety and nervousness, make a fog the dreaded terror of the sea (all the more terrifying because of its very silence and gentleness).[38]

If we control those fears as a mountain climber controls the fear of falling, we may gain from the strange solitude an imagined remoteness from the world that can be found only on the highest mountain tops—a feeling of pleasure and contentment that contrasts sharply with but joins a now repressed feeling of apprehension. The feeling is one of detachment from the realities of danger and a development of a new awareness, the result of a switching of perceptive and emotional gears. Bullough continues to clarify his concept:

> The working of Distance is, accordingly not simple, but highly complex. It has a *negative*, inhibitory aspect the cutting out of the practical sides of things and of our practical attitude to them and a *positive* side the elaboration of the experience on the new basis created by the inhibitory action of distance.[39]

Within Bullough's concept of distance and its inhibitory action, mastery occurs in the ability to remain semi-detached from the conflict and stress. At times, during the crescendo of anxiety and impending tragedy, mastery for the maintenance of distance becomes imperative. If this detachment were absent, the tension factors would prevent continued exposure to the art form. With the aid of "psychical distance" the tragedy becomes less personal, less intimate. Distance permits participation with disturbing concepts that ordinarily would be unacceptable. We can participate with the artist's work as art and not as reality. Bullough suggests, "What is most desirable is the utmost decrease of Distance without its disappearance."

Edmund Burke also understood the need for distance although he did not clarify it as did Bullough. He stated, "terror is a passion which always produces delight when it does not press too close…."[40]

These complex patterns of thought are absent in the face of direct real tragedy. No pleasure arises in the sight of the emaciated starving child in North Africa. The intimacy with reality does not permit psychological detachment, but there is the potential of a subtle pleasure when elicited through the dramatic process of the arts.

Summary

Let us return to the biological forces of self and species preservation and reiterate, so to stress, two aspects within these forces that are related to the enjoyment of the arts.

Human beings are biologically programmed, as is the mother bear for example, to nurture and protect our young, sometimes to the point of sacrificing self in our love of our young; a love that for human beings assumes significance in the arts.

We are also programmed to be gregarious, an aspect of our nature that is akin to the biological pattern of the wolf pack and the gazelle. There is safety in numbers and a greater chance of obtaining food since we cannot run, pounce or bite as the tiger. We need to hunt or work as a group. The possible precursor of Homo sapiens, the Homo habilis of East Africa had to live in a group, had to form attachments within the group in order to survive.

The feelings of love of our children, the reciprocal love of children to parents, the love toward our mate and the attachments, hot and cold, we develop with our fellow human beings, all become entwined with the myriad of sounds and sights that impinge upon us during the maturation of these feelings. These feelings become densely interwoven within the fabric of memory.

As we listen to music, watch dance, look at a painting, hear poetry and study drama, the reactions we feel are directly tied to this sturdy network of memory; a tie that impacts our reaction to all the arts although we may be unaware of their presence or their impact.

In essence, the mechanisms through which the arts incite emotion are fundamentally biologically driven, but markedly modified, enhanced, amplified, and controlled, or disciplined by the forces of acculturation. These forces may be so strong as to hide or to completely negate the basic animalistic impulses within us.

Chapter Four

A Definition of Aesthetics

Prior to the eighteenth century, literature (poetry and prose), music, dance, and the visual arts (painting, sculpture, and architecture) were discussed as separate entities, or under broad general categories of crafts, imitative arts, poetics, and beauty. Wladyslaw Tatarkiewicz describes this tradition.

> Hugh of St. Victor's classification of the arts, the most complete to be compiled during the Middle Ages, isolated the...sciences, and mechanical arts,...but made no provision for the fine arts. Nor did medieval thinkers set the fine arts above the other arts: when they had to name the higher arts, they mentioned only the liberal, or theoretical, arts. Of what we would call "fine art," music alone was considered as a liberal art. Architecture was included among the mechanical arts; painting and sculpture...were treated as crafts...the poet ceased to be a seer, but he retained his stature since poetry was included in the category of...knowledge.[1]

This disjointed categorization of the arts persisted despite the vast amount of study devoted to their different forms. The arts were not combined into a single cohesive unit until the philosopher Alexander G. Baumgarten (1714–1762) tied them together under a single heading when he used the word "aesthetics" in his discussion of art and its relationship to sensory knowledge. The word "aesthetics" is derived from the Greek word aesthetikos meaning of or pertaining to aisthita, things perceptible by the senses. Baumgarten's use of the word aesthetics not only unified the arts, but more importantly, implied the existence of a common denominator involving all the arts. This was a remarkable concept.[2] The subsequent acceptance of the term "aesthetics" and the implied unification of arts under a generic heading was a milestone in the study of the arts.

Although I assume that Baumgarten had an intuitive understanding that these subjects had a common bond, this common denominator was not and has still not been clearly defined. As a result, some scholars doubt that the various art forms have any quality in common.

Clive Bell vigorously attacked the problem of a common denominator of the arts. His effort was directed toward seeking a unifying element within the work of art itself. In his reference to the production of aesthetic emotion, he stated:

> if we can discover some quality common and peculiar to all the objects that provoke it, we shall have solved what I take to be the central problem of aesthetics….There must be some one quality without which a work of art cannot exist….What is this quality? What quality is shared by all objects that provoke our aesthetic emotions? What quality is common to…Mexican Sculpture, a Persian bowl, Chinese carpets, Giotto's frescoes…and Cezanne? Only one answer is possible—significant form.[3]

He then defines "significant form" as "…arrangements and combinations that move us in a particular way…."[4] But Bell does not define what is meant by "particular way," nor does he clarify "arrangements and combinations."

Theodor Adorno also stresses the idea of "form," referring to it as "…the sum total of consistency in art works and that …form is *the* distinguishing concept of art…," but then he admits that "There are difficulties when it comes to saying just what form is."[5] Susanne K. Langer comments that "Significant Form"…is the essence of every art. It is what we mean by calling anything artistic" and suggests we "…look upon the art object as something in its own right, with properties independent of our prepared reactions…."[6]

The approach of Bell, Adorno, and Langer that looks at the source for the common denominator was bound to fail. The diverse sources of aesthetic pleasure, say in poetry, painting, or dance as well as the diversity of the types of art among different cultures, ranging from the art of the Maori to that of Colima culture to New Guinea art to French Impressionism suggests that such a search would be fruitless. The structure or segment of structure within a work of art that assumes "significance" to one person may be totally meaningless to another.

In view of the different art forms and extreme diversity among the different cultures of the world, there does not appear to be any more validity in speaking of "significant form" applied to the art work than "significant perception" applied to the perceiver.

A similar attempt to identify a common denominator within the perceiver would probably be fruitless as well. A stimulus that may produce a marked emotional reaction in one person may have no significant effect upon another.

The marked difference in response among individuals of the same society and especially among individuals of different cultures suggests that if a common denominator underlying aesthetics does exist, but is neither in the stimulus nor in the perceiver, it must be within the character of the relationship which develops between them. Through an understanding of the special qualities of this relationship and the nature of its effect we may hopefully find a common thread that ties the psychological makeup of the perceiver to the work of art. The character of this relationship permits the perceiver to develop an aesthetic reaction. While Bell, Adorno, and Langer focus upon characteristics of "form," I prefer to concentrate upon the uniqueness of the relationship between the art and the perceiver.

Emotional responses to the arts may range from extreme pleasure to extreme displeasure. Since the reaction can exist anywhere within the spectrum of emotion, it is probably irrelevant, as far as the common denominator is concerned, whether the emotion sensed is joy or anger, depression or exaltation. If we assume this to be correct, then the common factor in the relationship would have to be in an unusual or unexpected aspect of the relationship.

Since neither human emotion nor the potential of a work of art to incite emotion can be measured with any degree of accuracy, it will be necessary to resort to the following images to help clarify what I mean by an "unusual or unexpected aspect of the reaction."

When you are touched by a wisp of cotton so lightly that you are barely aware of the touch, a baseline touch-awareness relationship is established which is the minimal amount of pressure necessary to produce the earliest awareness of touch. This will vary with individuals depending upon their sensory threshold. Similarly, a stimulus that just begins to evoke an emotional reaction establishes the baseline emotional relationship. In both cases, the response is in proportion to the stimulus. If a stronger stimulus is applied, such as a slap, we would expect an intensified response. Although the reaction to a stronger stimulus would be different in intensity and quality than to the baseline stimulus, the reaction would still be *proportional* to the intensity of the stimulus.

In regard to the emotion-awareness relationship, an intensified response could result from a scene of a mother gently touching and fondling her child. This image will, in most perceivers, produce a feeling of tenderness, warmth, and an awareness of mother's love. Although this would be a heightened feeling, it would still be an expected reaction consistent with the image and therefore proportional to the stimulus.

If an artist portrays a mother and child in a manner that produces the same degree of reaction in the viewer that would have taken place if exposed to the actual image, the relationship would only fall into the category of direct proportionality and therefore reflect skill, but not artistry. But if the artist portrays the image of the mother so that the response produced is not only of the expected quality of tenderness but of additional qualities, such as an intense awareness of the helplessness of the child, or of overwhelming mother-love, or an unexpected intensity of tenderness, then the reaction of the perceiver to the art work would be considered beyond the level ordinarily expected from the sight of a mother fondling her child. This reaction would place the relationship into a special category of unexpected enhancement of emotion. The special category is characterized by a response that is more intense or desirably different in quality than what would ordinarily be expected.

The following examples clarify this special category.

If a person is exposed to brutal death during war, the emotion evoked would be quite intense. The stimulus would be of major magnitude, and the response would be directly proportional to it. Although it is almost inconceivable to assume that moments of anguish during actual war could possibly be equalled on canvas or in literature regardless of the talent of the artist, the artist may be able to broaden the impact. The artist may expand the significance of that anguish and the concept of war itself. He or she may express the frailty of people, the strange quirks of fate, the waste and injustices of life, or other concepts. By doing so, even though there would be a lesser degree of anguish, a broadening of the impact would occur, an addition of qualities possibly not sensed during the actual incident, and therefore beyond what would ordinarily be expected. This would elevate the relationship between the perceiver and the portrayal of war into this special category.

We may apply the same principle to poetry as we examine William Carlos Williams's poem "The Term."[7]

A rumpled sheet
of brown paper
about the length

and apparent bulk
of a man
rolling with the

wind slowly over
and over in
the street as

a car drove down
upon it and
crushed it to

the ground. Unlike
a man it rose
again rolling

with the wind over
and over to be
as it was before.

This sensitive poem imbues rolling brown paper with an unexpected animation, human-like feeling and sense of vitality. This is an impression that would not ordinarily be obtained by exposure to paper floating in the streets.

The unexpected enhanced reaction to a stimulus is the common denominator underlying all art forms. It is the result of an unusual aspect of the relationship that cannot be delineated, but whose effect can be described. The common denominator lies neither within the stimulus nor the perceiver, but in a unique relationship between them that results in such reactions. If this phenomenon is common to all reactions to art, its existence validates Baumgarten's effort to tie all art forms together under the umbrella of aesthetics as a generic term.

If this concept is valid, aesthetics may then be defined as

> the study of a unique relationship between a stimulus and a perceiver characterized by an emotional response that is intensified above, or of a quality different, from what would ordinarily be expected from the evocative stimulus.

We must qualify this understanding of the aesthetic relationship by including the element of social pressure. Although the relationship may be consonant with the definition of aesthetics, some relationships that are acceptable to the individual might be unacceptable to society. The highly structured concepts of morality and religion may forbid expressions considered to be unnatural, antagonistic to nature or to God, perverse, or simply generally repugnant, and therefore beyond "reasonable limits." Closely-knit social orders place restrictions upon some forms of expression. It would be quite impossible for an artist living in New England during its rigid puritanical period to create a statue with exposed genitalia. A fig-leaf cover would be mandatory. Fortunately, the attitudes of society slowly change toward greater freedom of expression. As a result, what may be considered perverse and socially unacceptable as aesthetic today may eventually be accepted and placed in the category of aesthetics. Aesthetic relationships are in some respects intimately bound to the vagaries of social attitudes, fads, and conservatism. Glen Wilson referred to this tendency to retain the status quo: "In our conservatism, some react against uncertainty and therefore reject the new or novel, which not only demands freedom of thought, but acceptance of ambiguity and therefore relative uncertainty. Conservatism prefers the more familiar, the certain, the status quo."[8]

The reaction to the work of art is the aesthetic reaction. It is purely subjective. The individual's aesthetic sense is that ability to respond to impulses directed toward inciting human emotion and thoughts. The aesthetic potential of the object or event can only be realized when it relates psychodynamically to the emotional makeup of the perceiver.

The question arises as to whether the reaction must be desirable to the perceiver. Do we have to like what we see or hear in order to develop or recognize an aesthetic relationship? Not at all. Personal likes or preferences are not mandatory in aesthetic relationships. In fact, the reaction may be one of dislike and dismay, despite the awareness of an aesthetic quality in the relationship. Hugo A. Meynell supports this concept. He suggests, "One does not need to get any pleasure out of a work of art to judge that it is good…appreciation of a work of art is ambiguous; it can amount either to enjoyment of it, or to judge that it is able to be enjoyed by others."[9]

Unfortunately, we usually do not separate our reaction to art from the dynamics that take place. We therefore tend to tie the value judgment "it is aesthetic" to the statement "I like it." They are not necessarily related. By stepping back and thinking dispassionately, we may become aware that a reaction is beyond what would ordinarily be expected, but at the same time wish to terminate the relationship if the impact also produces disturbing and unpleasant feelings. Paintings, dramatic plays or poems of tragedy and anguish, regardless of how they may incite emotion or produce insight into life, may be too disturbing for some to view or to read. Although they may recognize that the reaction is beyond what would ordinarily be expected, many people could not live with Goya's "Prisoner" or Picasso's "Guernica" in their home. This does not imply that the work is devoid of aesthetic quality, but only that it is less desirable to that specific person.

Traditionally, the use of the term "aesthetics" has been restricted to literature, music, dance, visual arts, architecture, and more recently photography. However aesthetics may even include political rallies where the dramatic techniques may elevate the event to a form of drama.

The examples that I have cited to illustrate "unexpected enhancement" all use as a frame of reference known concepts or recognizable ideas. Under these circumstances, the viewer is psychologically forced to accept obvious reference points and anticipate reactions which would have been expected as the basis for comparison. This was seen in the mother and child example and the poem by Williams.

But what is the basis used for comparison to determine if the reaction is "beyond what would ordinarily be expected" when exposed to a totally new experience? How can we evaluate our reaction to a remarkable new image, such as a microscopic view of the eye of a fly, for the first time? In such cases the uniqueness of the object is unexpected. The newness of the situation arouses interest and curiosity. Joseph Addison appreciated this relationship. He commented that "Everything that is new...raises a pleasure in the imagination, because it fills the soul with an agreeable surprise, gratifies its curiosity, and gives it an idea of which it was not before possessed."[10]

Emotional excitement is gained through this curiosity, but it may wane after we become familiar with the concept. The stimulus may subsequently have to be more significant than simply a reproduction. Does the pleasure due to intense interest in a complex mechanical device make it an aesthetic experience? Possibly so, but just because something gives pleasure does not make it art.

In regard to non-objective visual art, which by definition does not supply the viewer with a recognizable concept, the aesthetic relationship depends upon whether the balance, unique juxtaposition, texture, flow, and rhythm of the forms or colors presented result in an unexpected enhanced feeling. The ball placed on a colored background is only a ball on a colored background, but if placed in a position so harmonious with the size and the color of the background that we are suddenly aware of a sense of balance and controlled tension, then the image assumes new attributes beyond the mere existence of a ball on a colored background. An exciting display of fireworks, and most symphonic and chamber music may be considered non-objective works of art.

Random sounds may begin to assume new significance when placed in a rhythmic structure. When given variations in pitch and texture within a rhythmic form, the potential for significance as music becomes even more pronounced. The leap from meaningless sound to music may be quite short, and the jump from color and form to nonobjective art may be equally short.

When we attempt to recognize an aesthetic relationship, we must be aware of a pitfall. Repetitive exposure and subsequent familiarity to any of the art forms may result in sophistication and appreciation of a given level of creativity and performance. This may lead to the use of past levels of creativity and performances as frames of reference. All art which equals or surpasses the level of prior similar endeavors would be considered to be of aesthetic significance, while all art which fell below would be termed unaesthetic. Although this approach may be used to establish levels of aesthetic relationships, it should not be used as a basis for establishing the fundamental aesthetic validity of the art work. We would be in error to assume that Bach or Beethoven have aesthetic value while simple folk tunes do not.

Chapter Five

Definition of Art

Morris Weitz denies the possibility of defining art, since "If we actually look and see what it is that we call 'Art,' we will find no common properties—only strands of similarities."[1] He bases this approach upon Wittgenstein's discussion of the definition of a game which defies the possibility of finding a common denominator in games that would define a game. Nelson Goodman wisely states,"to say what art does is not to say what art is, but I submit that the former is the matter of primary and peculiar concern."[2] Although the approach of Weitz, Wittgenstein, and Goodman is valid in one sense, we may speak to the "matter of primary and peculiar concern" and "define" something not only by what is a constant part of that something, but by the consistent and unique effect of the action or function of that something. An example would be the definition of a mail carrier who may be defined by the effect of the action as one who delivers mail so that others may communicate with each other. The mail carrier may be a man or woman or even a trained dog. As no common denominator applies to all mail carriers except for their function and the effect of their function, so no common denominator applies to the objects of art except for their ability to participate in a peculiar relationship with a perceiver. The common denominator of all the arts lies within the function and effect of art. Within this framework, Erwin Panofsky defines art as a "Man-made object demanding to be experienced aesthetically."[3]

Prior to discussing a definition of art, we should discuss a work of art either as an integral part of its historical period and site of origin, or as it stands independent of its maker, its time, its origin, or its cultural base, in short independent of its anthropological significance—but only as an aesthetic object. John Dewey comments, "When artistic objects are separated from both conditions of origin and operation in experience, a wall is built around them that renders almost opaque their general significance, with which aesthetic theories deal."[4]

Dewey's comment is valid if we are to consider the "general significance" of the artwork, but this does not deny the possibility of its purely aesthetic significance: being timeless and independent of its cultural origins. To completely understand a Yoruba sculpture demands an understanding of the context in which the sculpture was made, but that same piece of sculpture can be seen as purely an aesthetic object. Such an approach separates "art" as an anthropological entity from art as an aesthetic entity. A basis exists for this separation.

Are the parameters of aesthetics different for every culture and period? I believe they are superficially but not fundamentally. Despite the tremendous dissimilarity between the ethnic art of New Guinea peoples and the fine art of Michelangelo, in one respect they are not as different as you might assume. The similarity that exists independent of its anthropological aspects is based on the fact that the fundamental psychological mechanisms underlying aesthetics are quite uniform throughout all human beings and are only colored by, but not totally dependent upon cultural differences. If we study the crocodile heads carved on the prows of New Guinea canoes, we may be impressed with their sleekness and anthropological significance until suddenly we are exposed to one carving that appears the same as those on other canoes but is quite different. That difference has transformed the anthropological object into an aesthetic object recognized as such by the natives and tribal chieftains. If we compare the many ceremonial carvings of a given African tribe with the superior carvings used by the chieftain of that tribe, the aesthetic difference between the two groups becomes readily apparent. The difference in sculptural quality between the strength and power of Olmec sculpture or the lyricism of Jaina ceramics, and the vast group of Pre-Columbian arts, becomes quite apparent to contemporary sophisticated art collectors who may be totally ignorant of the tribe's mythology or symbolism. The monumental quality of the Amlash bull or the bull in the Lascaux caves, so apparent to our twenty-first century eyes, was probably also apparent in the eyes of their makers. In essence those works of art considered of superior quality were and are recognized as such by both contemporary sophisticated art dealers and collectors a as well as by the leaders of erroneously titled "primitive" societies. With an appreciation of this commonality we can look at a work of art from the aesthetic point of view without any reference to its period, place of origin or maker.

Art must be a cohesive, complete, and integrated unit, but I disagree with Stephen C. Pepper's statement, "no detail can be removed or altered without marring or destroying the value of the whole."[5] I believe that slight changes in choreography, painting, or musical score may at times enhance the original work of art. Great composers and painters frequently discussed their work and sought the advice of fellow artists prior to its completion. Johannes Brahms approached the violinist Joseph Joachim for his advice before completing the Brahms Violin Concerto. Because it is now complete does not mean that further advice would not have been welcomed by the artist.

Art has been defined in many ways. I would like to define art in terms of either what it should accomplish or how it may accomplish it, and yet adhere to the words of caution of John Hospers, who spoke of the pertinence of a non-judgmental definition when he stated, "The definition should be neutral with respect to value. It is doubtful whether a...definition of road should distinguish good roads from bad roads."[6]

Probably the most prevalent understanding of what constitutes art or at least "fine art" was expressed by Tolstoy. He defined art as an activity by means of which one person, having experienced a feeling, intentionally transmits it to others, who in turn experience the same feeling.[7] This definition seems incomplete. To transmit a feeling does not necessarily imply that the recipient senses a feeling which is beyond what would ordinarily be expected. This definition would therefore not fulfill my criteria of aesthetics since art exists only when an aesthetic relationship appears, not simply when a feeling has been transmitted. The example of mother and child exemplifies this principle.

Art may be defined as the method or vehicle by which an aesthetic relationship is established. This occurs when the work produced establishes a relationship between a stimulus and a perceiver characterized by an emotional response that is intensified above a level, or of a quality different, from what would ordinarily be expected from the evocative stimulus.

Art comes into existence whenever an artist can enhance, intensify, clarify, or bring insight into the quality of an object, a concept, or a feeling. Anything less is only an attempt to create art. As expressed by Vincent Van Gogh, "It all depends on how much life and passion an artist is able to express…."[8] Paintings, Van Gogh adds, should "not be made to please a certain taste in art, but to express a sincere human feeling."[9]

Art is usually considered a product of people and not a product of nature, but if the product of nature is modified by the manner in which it is displayed it may become an object of art. A piece of driftwood that is artistically displayed may become an aesthetic image. The all natural sand and rock gardens of Japan reflect the exquisitely refined aesthetic sense of that culture's relationship to objects of nature.

Science describes an entity or concept that may be intriguing and awesome. Art applied to that entity or concept reveals the potential of that entity or concept to be emotionally significant beyond their original effect. Theodor Adorno comments: "In every work of art something appears that does not exist."[10] That "something" is an amplification and modification of the real or imagined world, a clarification of the complex and the exposure of the essence of who we are and what we feel.

Nelson Goodman approaches this question from a different point of view. Instead of asking the question, "What is art?" he asks, "When is Art?", This is an interesting and valid approach as exemplified in his comment that a Rembrandt painting used as a blanket is simply a blanket and not a piece of art.[11]

The essence of aesthetic evaluation revolves around its ability to produce an exaltation or enlightened elevation of human feeling, the ability to extend the concept of the pleasing to that of the beautiful, to give tenderness an intensified sense of poignancy, to incite our curiosity, to transform simple phenomena to the awe-inspiring, all or any of which culminates in an incitement of feeling leading to empathic intimacy. Van Gogh suggests the identical concept. He stated:

> I can still find no better definition for the word art than art is man added to nature, reality, truth, but with a significance, a conception, a character, which the artist brings out in it, and to which he gives expression....[12]

Art, by the force of its impact, sharpens perception. Beethoven suggests that the isolating principle of art is that it tends to overcome and control our own mind, so that it will set forth the revelation.[13] This demands active participation by allowing the imagination to be provoked and incited, not only to be receptive, but to deliberately try to see, hear, and feel. In the process, art enhances our ability to sense and to feel; it enhances our perceptive acuity and our understanding and insight into life. Melvin Rader expresses it as, "Art is...fundamental to the whole enterprise of living as a means of expression, creation, and appreciation."[14]

There is a spiritual quality to art and especially to music. Sound exists in nature. Music is the soul of sound. George Steiner suggests that the spirituality that permeates all aesthetic works reflects the "real presence" of God. He states, "music and religious feeling have been virtually inseparable," and he refers to Yeats's comment, "No man can write Shakespeare, Homer, Sophocles, who does not believe with all his blood and nerve, that man's soul is immortal." Steiner then supports his discourse by paraphrasing Yeats: "no man can read fully, can answer answeringly to the asthetic, whose 'nerve and blood' are at peace in skeptical rationality."[15]

This approach of Steiner and Yeats carries the implication that the agnostic or atheistic scientist whose life-work is tied to "skeptical rationality," who questions and doubts everything, who lives in a state of hopeful skepticism, is unable to sense and appreciate the ethereal, ineffable transcendental feeling generated by a Schubert quintet. This inability of the theist to recognize the aesthetic potential of the rationalist lies in an unawareness of the spiritual similarities between science and religion.

What do I mean by this? The secularist's spirituality is that feeling of awe in the mystic grandeur of life gained through an intimate sense of oneness with the forces underlying the breath of life, the movements of the cosmos, and the unknown. Secular spirituality is nourished by the awareness that within the forces that dwell in a single living cell may lie the key to all knowledge; that mathematical expressions, or another unknown type of expression, still hidden, underlie the fundamental expressions we know today; that a bond joins together the jet airplane, the growth of the strawberry, and the speeding galaxies in time that is curved; that an equation fed into a computer may produce a sensual flaring line that reveals the rhythm and hidden beauty that lies within a formula of numbers; that an awareness of the movements within an atom establishes a bond of vitality between the animate and the inanimate. For the secularist steeped in "skeptical rationality," this awareness of the oneness and grandeur of nature leads to a feeling like reverence, a spirituality associated with the realization that we are part of a grand design. The belonging, the empathy, the oneness is with all of life, or rather all of nature, animate and inanimate. Secularists grasp the oneness of nature through reason rather than through faith. Their spirituality and awe result from an awareness of the complexity and simplicity of life lying within this oneness.

The feelings of the pious, whose spirituality is gained through the intense belief of the oneness as a pattern of God, and the rationalist tend to converge. Their paths toward the awesome are different, though their sense of oneness and their spirituality are similar. What truly separates them is that the secularist is much lonelier than the theist. "Skeptical rationalists" cannot speak to nature and the unknown as the pious can to God. "Skeptical rationalists" cannot hope for the hand of solace to caress their shoulders, nor can they see, as the pious can, death as a celebration in its homecoming to God's embrace.

Chapter Six

The Beautiful, the Sublime, and the Ugly

Beauty

In a conversation that took place about 430 B.C.E. between Hippias of Elis and Socrates, Hippias assumed that Socrates had asked him, what is beauty and what is it whose added presence makes other things beautiful?[1]

Two thousand five hundred years later, these questions still remain unanswered. Historically, beauty was the central theme in studies of art. This was so prominent that when "aesthetics" was applied as a generic term to the "fine arts," it was subsequently commonly defined as the philosophy of beauty. However, after numerous students of the arts failed to reasonably define beauty, this strong tie changed and beauty was slowly relegated to a secondary position in philosophic discussions of the arts. Jerome Stolnitz expressed this change:

> 'beauty' has receded or even disappeared from contemporary aesthetic theory…the generic value-term, 'beauty' has been replaced by some such locution as 'aesthetic value.' It is in the discussion of aesthetic value that "beauty" gets more attention, but even here it is only one among other value-categories, and its statement is fairly perfunctory.[2]

The repeated failures to successfully define beauty discouraged further attempts to do so to a point that Harold Lee stated, "It will always remain vague because beauty is a word rich in poetic and literary connotations." He suggested that beauty "is best used to denote only a part of the general field of aesthetic value, and that part need not be carefully delimited, but can be left more or less vague."[3] Theodor Adorno states that "Beauty cannot be defined…."[4] This attitude persists and the meaning of "beauty" has remained nebulous.

What interfered with our ability to define the term "beauty" was a concept inherent within Socrates' question. His question may be interpreted as suggesting that beauty is a function of a specific form or pattern within the object, that something exists which if added to the object would make it beautiful, something that may serve as a common denominator within all objects of beauty. If the question is analyzed in these terms, the object assumes primary importance. On this basis, Plato concluded that what is beautiful always reflects unique measurable proportions in its construction.[5] If this emphasis upon the object were true, what would be beautiful to the Western mind would also be beautiful to all societies, primitive or sophisticated, literate or illiterate. This is not always so. The implication that beauty resides within the object persisted for centuries and became a major source of confusion. It relates to our prior discussion regarding the place of the common denominator in all art.

Both Francis Hutcheson (1694–1746) and Archibald Alison (1757–1869) realized that such a common denominator could not exist, that beauty cannot be a function of the object independent of the perceiver. Hutcheson commented:

> Beauty…is not…any quality…in the object…without relation to any mind which perceives it….Were there no mind with a *sense* of beauty to contemplate objects, I see not how they could be template objects.[6]

Alison stated that any attempt to find properties common and peculiar to beautiful objects is "altogether impossible."[7] However, during this same period in history there is a vague suggestion in the remarks of both Edmund Burke (1729–1797) and Immanuel Kant (1724–1804) that they believed properties exist specific to what is beautiful. Burke implied the existence of a common denominator underlying beauty when he said, "I never remember that anything beautiful…was ever shewn, although it were to be a hundred people, that they did not all immediately agree that it was beautiful."[8]

Kant defined beautiful as "that which, apart from concepts, is represented as the object of a universal delight."[9] Use of the word "universal" suggests that what is beautiful is there to be recognized. If beauty is not sensed when it is sensed by the elite, that it only reflects poor taste on the part of the beholder. Kant did not identify the properties of beauty. Some students of visual art still believe that there are specific and universal properties in an object that establish the presence of beauty. In the area of music, Albert Schweitzer implied a correlation between specific music forms with specific emotions.[10] In his discussion of Beethoven and Bach, he referred to Bach's "...capacity for characterizing the various nuances of an emotion...." This implication that there is a feeling within, or a specific significance to a given form, supported the attitudes of Burke and Kant as well as Carroll C. Pratt's point that "music sounds the way emotions feel."[11] Neither music nor any art form contains emotion. They only awaken what lies within the individual. The feelings triggered into existence are dependent upon the make-up of the perceiver and his or her relationship to the work of art.

Although the concept of Burke, Kant, and Schweitzer that there is a factor within the object that allows the object to be beautiful, is erroneous, it appears to have a certain validity. What suggests that it is credible?

The fundamental emotional structure of all human beings, regardless of race or culture, is quite similar. If all people were as untouched as the newborn child, uncontaminated by the influence of diverse cultures, we could then assume that certain patterns inherent within the work of art could universally arouse pleasure and be similar for all people, but even this would vary with each individual due to genetic threshold differences. Although cultural patterns will vary between different societies, within any given society the mores, the cultural influences, are quite uniform. Since the basic emotional structure is similar and the cultural input within a given society is fairly homogenous, there will be a relative unanimity of tastes and attitudes, resulting in a similarity in response to any given art form *within that specific society*. The psychological studies of Max Schoen support this concept of societal sameness:

> in general, a musical composition not only produces a change in the existing affective state of the listener, but that its effect upon a large majority of the members of an audience is uniform to a striking degree.... No two people are affected exactly the same by any stimulus. This study shows, however, that a given musical selection will arouse a certain definite re-

> action and will arouse the same reaction in different occasions, in a large proportion of those who listen.[12]

This unanimity, or societal sameness, was the nucleus underlying the concept of Burke, Kant, and Schweitzer, although they did not express it as such. The sameness becomes much less apparent when different cultures are compared, except for elements that are directed specifically toward arousing primal emotional reactions common to all people, at which point a cross-cultural similarity of response may well occur.

Let us return to the problem of beauty. What do we mean by beauty? Can we define it so that it can apply to all cultures despite their diversity?

Part of the problem in defining "beauty" lies in its relationship to the "good." Etymologically, "beauty" is derived from the Latin, "bellus," meaning pretty, handsome. "Bellus" in turn is possibly a derivative of "benulus," a diminutive form of "benes," which is derived from "bonus," meaning good. Therefore, etymologically, the concept of beauty is probably related to the concept of good. The Middle English word "bealte" and the French word "beauté" are similarly related.[13]

The relationship of beauty to "good" is also expressed in the ancient Greek word for beautiful, "kalos," which is the word for virtue.

Regardless of its philological origin and its apparent tie to the concept of good, the definition of beauty must be approached from the base of common usage and general inference. We must be aware of the problems of common usage. A death-dealing cancer may be a beautiful tumor to a physician with a narrowly focused eye; a precise swing of a golf ball is commonly referred to as a beautiful movement; a crushing blow to the face of a boxer becomes a beautiful hit; and the heart-rending feelings aroused during a tragic play are also designated as beautiful. Susanne K. Langer is inclined to use the word in an equally broad manner.

> Every good work of art is beautiful....Beautiful works may contain elements that...are hideous...the emergent form, the whole, is alive and therefore beautiful, as awful things may be as gargoyles...and the Greek tragedies of incest and murder are beautiful....Beauty is expressive form.[14]

This does not say much. Vomit is also "expressive form." This broad use of the word "beauty" is gracefully accepted by society. But should such imprecision be accepted?

Despite its ethereal character, I would like to state the elements in a relationship involving beauty and to define it as a function of those elements. Beauty, as with any aesthetic concept, appears to be neither a component of an object nor an attribute within the perceiver, but a value, a function, of a specific relationship between them.

This relationship consists of three elements. The first is the presence of a pleasurable response. The second element is the absence of any unpleasant component in the relationship. What is beautiful is not only highly pleasurable but *purely* pleasurable. Relationships that contain elements of displeasure would not fall into the category of the beautiful as I define it despite the development of gratification or pleasure. Any aspect of art that reflects tragedy, pathos, anguish, forlornness, fear, sadness, or any similar quality, as so often expressed in Shakespeare, Goya, de La Tour, may effect emotion tremendously, may result in pleasure, and may be of major aesthetic significance, but would not be categorized as beautiful but rather as awesome, sublime, magnificent, grand and so forth.

The third element underscores the definition of aesthetics, namely, a response beyond what would ordinarily be expected. To establish this we must separate the merely pleasurable from what is beautiful. Although this separation cannot be sharply demarcated, when the pleasurable assumes the value of beautiful, a qualitative change occurs in feeling that is recognizable.

What are those qualitative changes?

There is an immediacy to it. Edmund Burke suggests that it "demands no assistance from our reasoning; even the will is unconcerned...."[15] Kant expressed the same thought in a slightly different manner. What is beautiful as separate from simply pleasurable or agreeable, "pleases immediately."[16]

As a result of the immediacy, an element of surprise is created that arouses curiosity. The combination of immediacy and curiosity produces a sharpened awareness of the stimulus, a more intense focus upon it and therefore a honed perceptive acuity. Due to the intense awareness, other thoughts fade. The result is a purity of feeling, a new emotional and cognitive clarity. In a circular or rebound fashion this clarity lends further impetus to perception. The result is an intensification of both the pleasure and the cognizance of the pleasurable phenomenon. *We become strongly aware of being aware.* We not only sense the beauty but rush to sense it more. With this intensified awareness, if strong enough, we become enveloped by it, imbued with a sense of intimacy and empathy. Beauty not only incites our emotions but grasps them.

Although the above wording may exaggerate the usual response to beauty, by the use of such language the psychodynamic play may be better understood.

The Dutch writer Frans Hemsterhuis (1721–1790) was aware of this unique intensity. He believed that beauty, which gives most pleasure, allows the greatest number of perceptions per unit time and therefore it is the highest cognition human beings can obtain.[17] Although I do not agree with this statement, since sudden threat to life may supersede beauty as producing "the greatest number of perceptions per unit time," it does support the concept of being "strongly aware of being aware."

Beauty, as I define it, being purely pleasurable, must be fundamentally based upon either the primal mechanisms of sexuality or curiosity. Freud's belief that "Beauty and attraction are first of all the attributes of a sexual object,"[18] tends to ignore the importance of the non-sensual sources of pleasure derived from curiosity: intense fascination.

Using the three elements—incitement of pleasure, pure pleasurableness (therefore no element of fear, tension or anxiety), and pleasure beyond what would ordinarily be expected; beauty may be defined as

> an intensified pleasurable relationship that is more than what would ordinarily be expected, devoid of any element of displeasure, and that results in an unusual sense of intimacy with the stimulus.

Expressions of art which contain elements of displeasure could not, within the narrow framework of this definition, fall within the category of beautiful.

Through the recognition of these factors, beauty may be recognized intellectually after being sensed emotionally. We recognize beauty through its effect. We are aware of being aware. We begin to understand it after "dispassionate" analysis of the characteristics of the emotion felt.

Guy Sircello suggests:

> we ultimately enjoy beauty because in perceiving beauty we seem to be better off than merely very well off. For in perceiving beauty we seem to be perceiving with a much greater degree of clarity than our ordinary clear perception has. In perceiving beauty we are filled, if only for a moment and if only in a limited respect, by a feeling of transcendent well-being.[19]

The object that participates in this relationship may be referred to as being beautiful. The degree of the perceiver's ability to participate may be considered the individual's sense of beauty.

What is beautiful always joins the realm of aesthetics since it is beyond what would ordinarily be expected or considered simply pleasing. But since beauty is limited by the absence of elements causing displeasure it must stand under the umbrella of aesthetics rather than alongside it.

The Sublime

Commonly associated with the word "beauty" is the word "sublime."

The definitions of sublime whether from the Oxford English Dictionary, Webster's Dictionary, or the American Heritage Dictionary, all have one element in common: what is sublime is lofty, grand, majestic, in essence, qualities that are appropriate to the Latin origin of the word *sublimis*, which means uplifted.[20] The Oxford English Dictionary refers to sublime in nature and art as "affecting the mind with a sense of overwhelming grandeur, or irresistible power; calculated to inspire awe, deep reverence, or lofty emotion, by reason of its beauty, vastness, or grandeur."

George Santayana speaks of the values in the beautiful as being "all positive" and the sublimely beautiful as being

> intoxicatingly beautiful...reaching such an intensity that it begins to lose its objectivity...,and to declare itself...an inward passion of the soul...in the sublime we find a purer and more inalienable perfection...that carries

> us away from the blurred objects before us, and raises us into a sort of ecstasy.[21]

If we use the concept of beauty as previously described, it may be of interest to discuss, as an example, the pleasure of a magnificent sunset and explore whether it falls within this understanding of the beautiful and the sublime. But first it is pertinent to cite Bendetto Croce's wise statement that "we must leave writers and speakers free to define the sublime...as they please and as may suit the end they have in view."[22] But Croce goes on to suggest that the word "overwhelming" is probably appropriate in use of the word sublime although still not quantified.

If the sunset makes us feel a delicate softness, lusciousness, and warmth, all sensations which are purely pleasurable, the relationship may be considered delightful, wonderful, but still not necessarily beautiful. But if the color and conformation of the sun and adjacent sky is *unusually* magnificent, beauty may be appropriate. If the feeling is associated with a sense of grandeur and exaltation, then a third element, the sublime, comes into play. Sublime may give to beauty a transcendental quality, an overwhelming feeling of intimacy with the beautiful. The beautiful may become sublimely beautiful. The sublimely beautiful is an extension of the beautiful, the highest level of the beautiful.

Robin G. Collingwood states:

> Sublimity is beauty which forces itself upon our mind, beauty which strikes us as it were against our will and in spite of ourselves...the shock of sublimity is the shock of an uprush of imaginative energy within ourselves....[23]

What is beautiful may be, but is not always, sublime, and what is sublime may be beautiful. But if the feeling of grandeur associated with the sunset is tinged with a feeling of and an awareness of our smallness, insignificance, insecurity, and subtle fear of the unknown, then it is no longer a question of beauty since within the definition of beauty a relationship that involves fear or any other form of displeasure may not be considered part of the beautiful. We are then left with sublime. This alternative becomes much more obvious when applied to tragedies in drama, literature, or in the visual arts where apprehension, tension, and fear are an intimate part of the experience.

This approach to the "sublime" is contrary to the thinking of Edmund Burke who evaluated sublime quite differently. He divorced it from its origin and from any relationship to beauty. Burke commented:

> terror is in all cases whatsoever, either more openly or latently the ruling principle of the sublime....The idea of the sublime and the beautiful stand on foundations so different, that it is hard, I had almost said impossible, to think of reconciling them in the same subject...[24]

Croce recognized that Burke derived the beautiful from the instinct of sociability and the sublime from the instinct of self-preservation.[25] This evaluation was based upon Burke's comment:

> The passions which belong to self preservation, turn on pain and danger; they are simply painful when their causes immediately affect us; they are delightful when we have an idea of pain and danger, without actually being in such circumstances; this delight I have not called pleasure, because it turns on pain, and because it is different enough from any idea of positive pleasure. Whatever excites this delight, I call *sublime*."[26]

Burke's attempt to separate sources of enjoyment derived from purely pleasurable sources and those derived from sources which contain elements of pleasure and displeasure is pertinent, but he did not appreciate the generic aspect of "pleasure," the various types of pleasure, some derived from self-preservation influences whereby pleasure may be associated with or derived from displeasure, and some from species-preservation influences. Using Burke's definition of sublime would suggest that the pleasure obtained from masochism and sadism would be sublime.

Alexander Gerard separated beauty from the sublime but did appreciate that both were pleasurable.[27] Kant believed that the idea of sublime may be best noted in the wild chaotic disorder and desolation of nature if it impresses one with a sense of great magnitude and power.[28]

In view of both its accepted usage and its origin, the term "sublime" should be limited to those aesthetic relationships which not only have the power to give pleasure but which have an uplifting quality to them.

Aesthetics, as a generic term, therefore encompasses three different pleasure-producing relationships:

1. the beautiful, composed of purely pleasurable elements,
2. the group with mixed elements of pleasure and displeasure of which there are varying proportions of both elements, and
3. the sublime which can be an extension or extrapolation of any of the first two categories if the relationship is awe-inspiring, uplifting, or overwhelming.

A specific word to express the second category is yet to be coined.

The Ugly

What is the place of ugliness in a discussion concerning aesthetics? Does it even belong in this area of thought?

If we assume, as some theologians may, that ugliness does not exist since all creation is the product of God, and the mind of God does not harbor any ugliness, then we must stop, for only a mathematician can meaningfully discuss what does not exist. On the other hand, if we are less inclined to look at life in such terms, we can assume that ugliness does exist. If so, what do we mean by "ugly," and what is its relationship, if any, to aesthetics?

As to its place in aesthetics, both the ugly and beautiful are related to emotion along the pleasure-displeasure spectrum. Since it may be of value to understand the total spectrum, both concepts should probably be studied under the umbrella of aesthetics. Stolnitz places the ugly within the study of aesthetics on the basis that "Ugliness designates aesthetic disvalue as beauty designates positive aesthetic value. The two therefore constitute a vague polarity…."[29] The ugly should therefore be part of the study of aesthetics if only to clarify this polarity.

What is ugly? As beauty is an intensification or extension of the purely pleasurable, so ugly is an intensification or extension of the purely unpleasant. They are both similar extensions in principle; therefore, they both fulfill the primary requirement within the definition of aesthetics as being "beyond what would ordinarily be expected."

Two reasons that prevent the ugly from being considered aesthetic is that such a relationship between perceiver and object may be either personally repugnant without any element of pleasure, or it may be socially unacceptable. But what ordinarily may be considered ugly could be portrayed so poetically that the image assumes aesthetic significance. An example of such a shift might be of the Hunchback of Notre Dame in which the physical ugliness of Quasimodo is tempered by the nobility and majesty arising from the exquisite tenderness and intensity of his love while faced with the impossibility of its fruition. Works of art which contain elements of the ugly may evoke gratifying feelings of some sort and therefore fall within the framework of aesthetics, as do works of art which contain elements of tragedy. But what is purely and only ugly, or purely and only tragic, without extenuating circumstances that give it a poetic quality, cannot fall under the umbrella of aesthetics. This is consonant with the comment of James L. Jarrett who states:

> A work of art is ugly when, although it attracts and even sustains aesthetic interest, it punishes rather than rewards that attentiveness: it signifies that the elements of painful aversion are too strong.[30]

Under these circumstances the work of art itself cannot be termed ugly, only that undesirable element, that if isolated from the total art effort, might be considered ugly.

Burke has related the ugly to the "sublime." He suggests that ugliness can become sublime when associated with strong terror. He stated, "Ugliness I imagine likewise to be consistent enough with an idea of the sublime. But I would by no means insinuate that ugliness of itself is a sublime idea, unless united with such qualities as excite strong terror."[31]

Burke's concept of sublime, in relationship to beauty, and the ugly, by invoking the element of terror, has divorced the word from its Latin origin "sublimis." Terror does not produce the sense of uplifting inherent in the word of its origin, "sublimis."

Chapter Seven

Psychological Aspects of Non-Objective Art

Non-objective art is art devoid of specified content. It is not an abstraction or summary of a given object but is form, space, movement, color, sound, or silence so constructed as to induce a specific feeling without any preset conditions.

Abstract art is art that is a summary or a derivative of realistic or figurative art. It lies between realistic and non-objective art. Abstract art is exemplified by the later art of Pablo Picasso and Marc Chagall as opposed to the non-objective art of Piet Mondrian and Jackson Pollock.

Poetry, prose, and musical forms which contain specified content, as in opera or songs, do not fall into the non-objective category. They are analogous to paintings with specified content as landscapes or portraits. But musical forms such as chamber music and symphonies, which usually are devoid of specified content, are analogous to non-objective visual art which contain form, color, and texture but are devoid of content in the sense of known object symbols. Dance divorced from preset themes is almost but not quite non-objective since the human body is so intimately involved. Although music may evoke images from memory, the image is not an integral part of the music except in the mind of that specific listener, it is not presented to the listener.

Non-objective visual art may be considered to be a visual form of non-objective music. A similar aesthetic basis and an equal aesthetic validity exists between non-objective art and art with content. The major difference between non-objective visual art and non-objective music, aside from one being visual and the other aural in character, is the element of time. Music may be more effective in its aesthetic impact since it carries over a relatively long time span compared to the usually short time spent in the experience of a non-objective painting or one with specified content. Experiments to elongate visual art in the manner of some Chinese and Japanese horizontal scrolls may be of interest.

Non-objective art is not chaotic. It expands the envelope to increase the potential for aesthetic relationships. In this respect. Mondrian, probably the greatest influence in non-objective visual art, correctly defines his subject: "Nonfigurative art is created by establishing a dynamic rhythm of determinate (a defined area in space)…relations which excludes the formation of any particular form…."[1]

Although he may be biased in his evaluation of its importance, Mondrian was so impressed with this tangent in art that when speaking of the evolution of art, he denigrated figurative art. In his terms,

> the culture of particular form is approaching its end. The culture of determined relations has begun….Precisely by its existence non-figurative art shows that "art" continues always on its true road. It shows that 'art' is not the expression of the appearances of reality such as we see it, nor of the life which we live, but that it is the expression of true reality and true life—indefinable but realizable in plastic.[2]

Mondrian did not appreciate the to-and-fro trends and movements within the arts over time. It was short-sighted, if not arrogant, to assume that future art of major aesthetic significance may not include a more figurative approach. The evolution of art is quite unlike the linear path of life from birth to death. Mondrian took a great leap of faith and portrayed a remarkable bias in his evaluation of non-objective and figurative visual arts.

The public's acceptance of non-objective visual art is generally much less than its acceptance of non-objective music. Why do the majority of people prefer visual art with content rather than visual art without content? We may better understand the basis for this difference if we appreciate a unique psychological difference between vision and hearing.

Almost all that we see in life is immediately impressed upon us in such a way that the potential for recognition becomes easy. Even though we may be unfamiliar with an object, we can almost always place it within a general category.

Joseph Addison in 1712 recognized this unique quality in sight. He commented, "Our sight…may be considered as a more delicate and diffusive kind of touch, that spreads itself over an infinite multitude of bodies, comprehends the largest figures, and brings into our reach some of the most remote parts of the universe."[3]

This does not hold true for sound. Most background sounds heard during the early formative period of life as well as in later life are devoid of intellectual or emotional significance and therefore are relatively meaningless. We are quite oblivious to the exact nature of sounds surrounding us since they tend to lack specificity. They usually remain uncategorized and vague as to their origin and exist only as an amorphous background. All too often, we are totally unaware of sound until it ceases, bringing into focus a delicious silence.

Because of our psychological detachment to unfocused sound, we neither consciously nor unconsciously demand that sound be recognizable. As a result, we can accept the sound of music without need to categorize it, and therefore we can more readily accept its non-objective character. But because of our ability to recognize and categorize all that we *see*, we unconsciously desire to retain this recognition-capability and are therefore uncomfortable and insecure in the absence of content.

James Ackerman spoke to this point when he referred to:

> the tendency we have to reform unfamiliar or unarticulated shapes in terms of everyday experience. The Rorschach Test, for example, is a successful diagnostic tool because nearly everyone is ready to interpret ink blots as representatives of things. Apparently it is an innate human tendency, at times a need, to organize visual data in terms of images from the raw material of everyday life.[4]

In view of this attribute of sight, unless the unconscious demand to recognize is lessened by exposure and training, the ability to participate with non-objective visual art may be difficult.

A negative aspect of non-objective art as exemplified by the work of Jackson Pollock, Mark Rothko, and Hans Hartung is that although pleasure may be obtained, insight, understanding, or empathy into the feeling or spirit of others or of nature may be difficult to reach. On the other hand, broadening of feelings or understanding is readily derived from art with recognizable content. The potential for an educative aspect to art that may enhance sensitivity that would be applicable to a broad spectrum of life necessitates recognizable content that may serve as the base upon which insight may flourish. There must be some new bit of knowledge, or further insight to what is already known, that expands the intellect. Poetry is a prime example. Visual art such as Millet's "Sower" may produce insight into the anguish and toil of poor farmers.

Although the educative factor in non-objective art is less than in figurative art, there is an educative aspect to non-objective art that is applicable to all the arts. As we listen to a Beethoven sonata, we will enjoy it to a certain level, but if we have the good fortune to be with a fine musician who can point out nuances of which we were not aware, our sensitivity, enjoyment, and appreciation of the music will be expanded. This increase in awareness and understanding of the music carries over to enhance our enjoyment of other music. We can learn how to listen and how to see.

There is an aspect of knowledge of the arts that can be detrimental. When we approach a work of art with rigid demands for a level of performance based upon prior experience, an unconscious resistance to its aesthetic impact may occur if the work is not quite as wonderful as the work with which it is being compared. In a different manner, the serious student of the violin may not enjoy a violin concerto as much as a non-student if too much of a conscious and unconscious tendency is present to evaluate technical nuances within the performance. This danger exists in all art-forms. Knowledge of the application of paint, the chemistry of paint, or the history of painting may unconsciously pull the psyche of the viewer to that area of knowledge. As a result he or she may not be psychologically free to fully enjoy the painting due to an inhibition of emotional play. But the greater the understanding the perceiver brings to the art-object, the greater that perceiver's potential to achieve maximum effect despite the danger of inhibiting emotional play through the conflict between intellect and emotion.

Another pitfall with knowledge is the tendency to overemphasize its importance. This is most common among those who never had a high degree of sensitivity to start with. This can lead to intellectual elitism superimposed upon a cold soul. I do not mean to say that knowledge is undesirable, on the contrary it allows us to better appreciate the nuances within art, but it can both help and hinder feeling. As it applies to the arts, we must seek knowledge, but not idolize it.

Chapter Eight

The Artist, the Perceiver, and the Aesthetics Lens

The Artist

The artist is endowed with an unusual degree of sensitivity and the ability to transmit poignant feelings via an art-form to incite emotion in others. He or she is able to penetrate beyond the obvious. The artist senses and separates the essence from non-essentials, intensifying, sharpening and clarifying that essence. Then, by focusing our thoughts and feelings, the artist enters our consciousness and unconsciousness with that insight. The artist may see a line or hear a chord, appreciate their emotion inciting potential, and translate that potential so that others may react. Talented artists do not merely incite a feeling but expose the mystery beneath and within it. They do not imitate nature. They expose its potential and convey its grandeur. The ordinary becomes extraordinary, while the essence of the complex and profound is revealed. The artist is endowed with an enlightened intuition.

These remarks may appear exaggerated if applied to the majority of artists, but when greatness is achieved, these attributes appear valid. J.W.N. Sullivan expresses this concept differently. He commented, "The great artist, painter, poet, or musician makes us aware as we have never been aware before. He extends and subtilizes certain elements of our experience and so gives us greater knowledge and mastery of life."[1]

Croce spoke to this principle in relationship to visual art when he stated:

> The painter is a painter because he sees what others only feel or catch a glimpse of, but do not see. We think we see a smile, but in reality we have only a vague impression of it, we do not perceive all the characteristic traits of which it is the sum, as the painter discovers them and is thus able to fix them on the canvas.[2]

When this has been accomplished, visual art in the true sense is created. This concept of art was also expressed by Vincent Van Gogh when he said, "a picture…says more, and says it more clearly, than nature herself,"[3] and again when he wrote of Millet's "Sower," "there is more soul than in an ordinary sower in the field." That is what art and aesthetics is all about, and reflects what must underlie all art-forms. The comments of Croce and Van Gogh reflect one of the remarkable attributes of the painter: a visual sensitivity, a conscious awareness of the details within an image. This ability to "see" may be enhanced through training, but it is primarily an inherent attribute of the artist.

Aside from the mystery of talent, in order for artists to accomplish their tasks he or she must be able to, at least partially, detach self from emotion. This may be most pertinent during the composition of music. The element of detachment was discussed by Roger Fry who said, "It is evident that the artist feels these emotions in a special manner, that he is not entirely under their influence, but sufficiently withdrawn to contemplate and comprehend them."[4]

The effort in creating a musical score or a painting is primarily an intellectual endeavor with minimal emotional input. The intensity of the noetic effort tends to push aside emotional input associated with the art concept, but does have emotional input during, and related to, the struggle to create. The emotional significance of the work is mainly sensed upon its completion.

John Dewey comments that during the act of producing with the intent to produce something of aesthetic significance, "The artist embodies in himself the attitude of the perceiver while he works."[5] his concept may not be entirely valid. I doubt that Picasso considers the public's attitude when he works. He does what he feels he must do to express his own thoughts. Dewey's comment raises the issue of societal attitudes and fads which may influence the direction the artist takes more than the artist's artistic judgment.

Richard Strauss went so far as to say, "I work very coldly, without agitation, without emotion even; one must be completely master of oneself to organize that changing, moving, flowing chess board orchestration."[6] Although Strauss's statement is not psychologically valid since it is quite improbable that we can separate cognition involving complex reasoning processes from emotion, it does suggest that what we feel when exposed to a work of art is not necessarily what is felt by the artist, nor does the work necessarily give insight into the artist's personality or character. The work of art is not truly the window through which we can see the heroic qualities of the artist as suggested by Thomas Carlyle. He commented:

> Find a man whose words paint you a likeness, you have found a man worth something; mark his manner of doing it, as very characteristic of him...he could not have discerned the object at all...unless he had...sympathized with it...a man without worth cannot give you the likeness of any object.[7]

These kind words belie the fact that an artist may have a character that would make a wolverine appear angelic and yet be capable of expressing the glory of life within a dying leaf.

What drives the artist? Multiple factors must underlie the act of creation, including simple enjoyment of the process. Some artists may be impelled to exploit their natural talent to avoid guilt in ignoring talent. Some may be impelled to create for the pleasure derived from the mastery of their craft, an impetus toward self-improvement. Some artists may be unconsciously impelled to create to resolve deep emotional issues and conflicts. Satisfaction may be gained from the discipline of achieving solutions to an artistic dilemma, the pleasure gained through mastery in achieving one's goal. A sense of élan may be experienced during the process of creating, and possibly ego satisfaction in the knowledge that one's work will be appreciated.

In the process of creativity lies an awareness of self-fulfillment, of personal growth. But if the artistic endeavor is constantly confronted by the difficulty of achieving a level of artistry anywhere near that of a Picasso or a Beethoven, the degree of constant frustration may be quite destructive. It may lead to an anti-establishment psyche that converts the artistic drive, that has aimed too high, to an attempt to be totally different, to stand out. It is very unlikely that a fine work of art will result if the artist's primary intent is to be different. Such attempts will tend to cast a shadow upon the integrity of the artist. Dispassionate intellectualization may become a prominent force at the expense of emotion and artistic integrity. Much of avant-garde art may be the result of this approach rather than the result of an artistic creative drive.

Artistry and artisanship are not synonymous.

The ancient Greeks referred to both works of art and craft as "techne," which does not refer to technique or the technical; instead, as Martin Heidegger explains, it "denotes…a mode of knowing. To know means to have seen in the widest sense of seeing, which means to apprehend what is present, as such."[8]

Art goes beyond flawless artisanship or great skill; it may even be independent of great skill. Artistry demands the ability to project the intensity and essence of whatever the artist perceives so that it may incite a unique emotional reaction in others, an emotional reaction beyond what would ordinarily be expected from the subject matter. This necessitates the existence of a talent that is different than the talent of a pure artisan, a talent that separates the creative artist from the talented artisan. Excellent artisanship does not necessarily produce art. This does not negate the dignity of skill but only separates it as an entity from art. Skill is needed to construct a table, but a table is rarely a work of art. If the worker can create a table which incites an unusual or unexpected degree of feeling, then that work may be art, and the artisan then falls into the category of artist as well as artisan. The technical skill necessary for artists to create is crucial to their creativity, but it is secondary to their artistic sense. The primary function of craft is utilitarian, while the intent of an artist is primarily to incite emotion, also a utilitarian endeavor, but less tangible.

Art and crafts are also separated by the difference in process. The artisan is fully aware of what the end result will be, the exact steps necessary to reach that goal, and a carefully laid out plan of attack that will prevent any errors. This is unlike the artist who tends to adapt to a new feeling or image and allows for a certain fluidity as the work progresses. An ambiguity usually persists throughout the process of creativity until the end has been reached.

The Perceiver

Throughout life, we consciously see, hear and feel primarily to serve our immediate needs. The arts do not serve our daily needs. They offer perceivers the opportunity to see and hear for the pleasure of what they perceive. We do not look at an office building with any special vision unless we look at it as an architectural form. With this new vision, our imagination is excited, our emotional substance enhanced, and our life is thereby enriched.

The character of the feeling response, the perceiver's reaction, is usually, but not necessarily the kind of reaction the artist believed would be sensed. The relationship is between the perceiver and the work of art, not between the perceiver and the artist, even though the work of art is a product of the feeling or thought that reflects the feeling or thought of the artist. Clive Bell states, "In pure aesthetics we have only to consider our emotion and its object: for the purposes of aesthetics we have no right, neither is there any necessity, to pry behind the object into the state of mind of him who made it."[9] Hugo A. Meynell paraphrases T.S. Eliot, saying that "the value of a work of art is not a function of the artist's intention...but of the disposition of the work itself to give satisfaction...."[10]

As the artist must have talent to conceptualize and transmit an idea with emotional impact, the perceiver must have the ability to respond, a degree of sensitivity, and, what is probably more important, a receptive attitude.[11] The ability to respond is not measurable and is as different for each person as is the fingerprint.

A perceiver's sensitivity potential is genetically determined, but although the capacity is fixed, the ability is expandable within the constraints of genetic limits and directly dependent upon the quality of life's impact. The enhancement and refinement of our sensitivity level is directly related to the degree and type of exposure to the arts. We can learn to see better, hear better, and "feel" better.

The perceiver must want to feel, to sense, to be willing to explore, to permit emotion to be tapped, to let oneself be psychologically immersed into whatever art form is presented, and to live fully within the moment, to reach, as Roger Fry expresses it, "disinterested intensity of contemplation."[12] The aesthetic attitude demands an open-mindedness and a desire rather than just a willingness to participate. Art does not reach out and tell you what to feel. You must make the effort to open widely its slightly ajar door. If the opportunity to participate is utilized, it allows the perceiver to achieve the greatest pleasure and insight possible from exposure to art regardless of its genre. Aesthetics demands active personal involvement. Unfortunately, some people lack the ability to allow themselves to be inwardly moved. Inhibitions and tensions may prevent a free flow of imagination or the amount of relaxation necessary to wholeheartedly participate in the art. In this respect, George Steiner's comment is of special interest and of great value. He suggests that "Accurate recollection and resort to remembrance…deepens our grasp of the work."[13]

A person may be well-endowed in one attribute and dismally lacking in others. He or she may have a capacity for deep sensitivity that has been undeveloped or may be highly trained and educated in the arts, yet lack sensitivity. A person without formal education may have an intuitive sense of major magnitude with an equivalent aesthetic sense.

On the other hand, the "expert" in the arts, although knowledgeable, may be aesthetically bland. This possibility should be appreciated. It would be a mistake to assume that art may be understood and appreciated only by the trained artist or scholar.

The Aesthetic Lens

Of major importance is the continuing development of the aesthetic attitude, an open receptive approach to the art form. This has significance far beyond the enjoyment of the arts. The aesthetic attitude becomes a lens, an aesthetic lens, which can enlarge our potential to enjoy all sensory input and therefore broaden our intellectual and emotional horizons. With this attitude, curiosity is enhanced and fostered. As a result, we can derive greater pleasure from the ordinary by seeing the ordinary with a broader and deeper vision. The mundane becomes intriguing, and the profound becomes more poignant. A chair is not only something to sit upon, but a dynamic form with ties to the romance of history. It is through the enhanced curiosity, the interest to be involved, and the insight given us through the use of the aesthetic lens that we can expand the depth and breadth of life. We can enhance our own understanding, we can see life in a different way with a different perspective, we can sense the awesome significance of dew, detect the hidden form in a rock, savor delicacy in snow, and gain a glimpse into life's grandeur. In essence, art allows us to grasp the potential emotional significance of all the forms and sounds that surround us. As William Blake put it in the "Auguries of Innocence,"

> To see a world in a grain of sand,
> and a heaven in a wild flower,
> Hold infinity in the palm of your hand,
> and eternity in an hour.[14]

Chapter Nine

Obligations Between the Artist and Society

The enrichment of our culture is strongly dependent upon the creativity of the arts. In the same vein, the development and productivity of artists, regardless in which genre they may work, is affected by the attitudes and responses of society. Artists do not work only for themselves. If no public existed, no art would exist, only doodlings. This reciprocal relationship demands recognition of the bond and the forces at play between artists and the public. The principle underlying and guiding this relationship is the self-interest of both groups. Appreciation of this force exposes the degree of mutual responsibility. Neither support of the arts, the production of art, nor artistic integrity are purely acts of altruism.

The most apparent consequence of the impact of art on the public is interestedness, a form of pleasure. But if this were the only effect of art, it would not be more important than any other source of pleasure. What is most crucial yet not obvious is the effect of art upon our sensitivity and our emotional awareness. That awareness tends to alter our approach to the commonplace object or event. Through the arts, our empathy toward the ordinary changes. A cat crossing the street becomes a rhythm of feline grace. The pot is not just a water container but an object of artistic engineering skill.

Part of the greatness of art and one of the most valuable by-products of art is the enhancement of human sensitivity and a broadening of our vision. In the awareness of suffering in drama, visual art, or literature lies an awakening of what is magnificent in life's struggle: the daydream, the impossible dream, the search for goodness, the poignancy in the frailty of man and woman, the nobility in striving for moral strength and loftiness of character, dignity achieved in the face of tribulation, awareness of human spirit which is capable of reaching great heights of compassion and sense of love, an affirmation that there can be tenderness, compassion and purpose in life despite the tragedy which is an integral part of life. Thanks to art, we can more easily appreciate the human will to live with a sense of purpose despite awareness of its insignificance in the grand pattern of the universe. Within nobility and the unconscious awareness of moral worth lies an understanding that life has direction and need not be a haphazard moment. This enhancement of our emotional foundation and perception widens our scope. The potential net result is the enrichment of all future moments of life with an ever-increasing frontier as well as a greater sense of living within the moment.

With this realization, we may appreciate the arts as a crucial need for the development of the human mind and not simply as a source of gratification. This concept is not sufficiently understood by either the artist or the public.

The Artist's Obligation to Society

The artist's obligation to society is in many respects identical to his or her obligation to self. I do not adhere to the Marxist approach that demands that artistic efforts be directed toward improving social patterns and conditions of the community. This does not mean that art that speaks to the tragic and unjust in life is not to be appreciated for its social effect, but the effort of the artist should be the result of an inner drive rather than the result of a social demand. Francisco Goya's "Fifth of May," Honoré Daumier's social satires, and David Siqueiros's magnificent murals all have important messages, but messages done freely, not as a result of a social demand imposed upon the artist.

The major burden placed upon the artist by society, and hopefully taken seriously by the artist, is maintenance of a high degree of artistic integrity despite society's apparent apathy to the arts. Society's dependence upon the arts is of such major significance that, in return for its support, it has a right to expect that the artist's sense of dedication to the arts will not be violated. Only the artist is in the position to recognize "artistic integrity." An outstanding example of artistic integrity in the field of painting was the action of Georges Rouault who destroyed many of his paintings that he considered were not of significant aesthetic value. Periodic critical re-evaluation with a more detached attitude would eliminate much art of mediocre quality and would more adequately portray the artist's aesthetic concepts.

Van Gogh reflected a similar sense of integrity:

> I have mercilessly destroyed one important canvas—a "Christ with the Angel in Gethsemane" and another one representing the "Poet against a Starry Sky" in spite of the fact that the color was right—because the form had not been studied beforehand from the model....[1]

Aside from maintaining artistic integrity, artists have an obligation to help society understand their work. This function, to a great extent, has been relegated to the critic. If this component of the artist's responsibility would be more thoroughly recognized, then the public would develop a more intimate understanding of artists and their problems and a greater rapport with the arts, thereby fostering a more widespread participation which would be of benefit to both the artist and the audience. The gulf between the creator and perceiver would narrow.

Society's Obligation to the Artist

Society's obligation to the artist is directed primarily toward the protection of the artist's creative sense, the enhancement of the artist's creativity, and enlargement of the public's opportunity for greater exposure to the arts for the direct benefit to society and to the artist.

Protection of the artist's creativity becomes an important issue whenever society tends to formulate guides or restraints concerning the artist's expression. This is dangerous in principle and in practice.

Aside from the immediate loss to society of a more diverse exposure, the limiting of artistic expression establishes a precedent that may permit further limiting concepts to be formulated, thereby engulfing and smothering the artistic essence. The periodic attempts by society to channel and restrict the direction of an artist's effort especially prevalent during moments of societal self-righteousness is reminiscent of the banning and burning of books by dictators. The pressure for artists to modify their work or their thoughts to satisfy their government, although subtle, is destructive. Dimitri Shostakovich's apology to the Kremlin for his music and Yevgeny Yevtushenko's revision of his poem "Babi Yar" for political reasons reflect the problem of governmental interference. One publisher's representative in the Soviet Union remarked to Arthur Koestler that "We build up the reputation of writers whom we think useful; we destroy writers whom we consider harmful; aesthetic considerations are petit-bourgeois prejudice."[2]

Fears that gross, crude, and vulgar statements may at times be detrimental to society are probably warranted, but the occasional unwise or socially unacceptable acts or statements by artists should not be used as an excuse for setting limitations. Restrictive actions in the long run, would create much greater harm to society than would any artist's work that might be considered undesirable to society. Such restrictions portray a lack of confidence in the ability of society to surmount transient cultural setbacks. Clive Bell remarked, "The more completely the artist is freed from the pressure of public taste and opinion...and the menace of words…the better for him and the better for art, and therefore the better for everyone."[3]

The problem of enhancing the work of artists revolves around the difficulty of enabling artists to devote sufficient time to foster their creative sense. This is an exceedingly complex issue. In our present social structure, artists frequently have great difficulty adequately maintaining their family while devoting full time to their art. This situation has been in existence for centuries despite the nostalgic frequent reference made to the patron-artist relationship prevalent during past centuries.

In the thirteenth to the eighteenth century, the prime support of the arts came from the limited few in political and financial power and from the church. During this period, such support was not a blanket subsidy for the arts, but was channeled to the support of specific artists, or specific schools led by those artists, while many desirous of such training or work were ignored and thereby forced to develop by their own efforts.

During those years, a well-established middle class did not exist. During the past centuries, a middle class of significant proportions has developed and has indirectly assumed the role of patron through the ability to purchase art and to afford concerts and theater. This development has not only eclipsed the isolated patron, but has given artists greater opportunity to develop since their work may now be seen or heard by a diverse population rather than depend upon the taste, desires, and opinions of a few.

This desirable diversification of support has its downside.Has a broad base of diverse tastes been an influence in the development of high aesthetic concepts, or has it been a force in developing the public's willingness to accept mediocre work as a statement of high aesthetic significance? Despite the potential downside, middle class support of the arts is a move in the right direction similar to governmental support of research, much of which fails to be of significant value.

The amount of fine talent that has never been allowed to flourish due to lack of educational opportunities must be immense. The flowering of talent among the African-Americans during the past twenty years due to greater opportunities is an indication of what had been lost to history in earlier decades.

Chapter Ten

The Critic

Criticism of the arts as a profession or avocation existed as long as there were arts to condemn or applaud. In "The Iliad" is a detailed critique of the artistry of Hephaestus as he meticulously fashioned a glorious shield for Achilles.[1]

In past centuries, although philosophers, artists, and students of the arts wrote about the arts it was a sporadic effort primarily reaching the intellectual elite. With the progressive development of print and the broadcast media in line with population growth, larger segments of the population were progressively introduced to the arts, reaching its peak during the twentieth century with the advent of expanding newspapers, radio, and television. Today, the "art critic" has carved a distinct niche in the social fabric of society.

The relationship between the critic, the artist, and society has been marked by dissension. This is due to the impression of large segments of the population that critics usually do not fulfill a valuable role for the artist or the public and therefore do not deserve the status granted them by society. The manner in which many critics react to the artist's work reflects a certainty of their impression whereby they deliberately or inadvertently assume the unwarranted position of taste definer. A critic's unfavorable review of a play may doom that play.

The critic has multiple functions. He or she must be an historian, a technical expert, and an aesthetician.

As an historian, the critic should understand the pattern of evolution of the art form, the significance of its relationship to the political, economic and attitudinal changes in society both old and new, the historical significance of support by royalty and the church as opposed to present day support by consumers after the work has been completed, the personal trials and tribulations of the artist and their effect upon the art work, and the debt the artist may owe to prior artists, such as Bach's debt to Vivaldi, and Picasso's debt to African sculpture.

As a technician, the critic should understand the technical aspects of the art-form whether it be the harmonic progressions in a musical score, the violinist's use of an up-bow instead of a down-bow, the painter's concept of perspective or the nuance in a pas-de-deux. In view of the complexity of each art form specialization becomes a necessity. The critic with knowledge and understanding of visual arts is not necessarily capable of functioning as a music critic.

It is the critic's role as an aesthetician that I believe is the critic's most important function.

The public listens to the critic for several reasons, but I believe the most important reason is to help them understand and enjoy the artist's work. This demand upon the critic is a heavy burden that unfortunately is rarely fulfilled. For critics to fulfill this function they must be endowed with a strong perceptive sense, high sensitivity, considerable intelligence, and a firm grasp of the historical and the technical aspects of the specific art form.

The critic should have the ability to express to others the poetic nature of the work. This demand places the "true" critic close to the poet. Unfortunately, we are linguistically stymied when driven to express what we feel upon exposure to the arts, especially to music. The English language is inadequate to express all nuances of emotion. It is unlike the indirect Japanese language where syllables within a word may have emotional nuances. Hopefully, extensive experience has honed the critic's sensitivity and language facility, and has enabled the critic to compare different works to help elucidate the concept he or she wishes to express.

George Steiner comments that the truest critic is the performing artist as reflected in the attempt to bring out the most meaningful aspect of the work regardless of whether it is a musical score or a dramatic text.[2]

The critic must examine what incites our interest and emotion; what makes the artist's effort a work of art. Otherwise, as stated by Clive Bell:

> If they are not curious about the nature of their emotion nor about the quality (in art)...that provoke it...let no one suppose that what they write and talk is aesthetics....A good critic may be able to make me see in a picture that had left me cold things that I had overlooked, till at last, receiving the aesthetic emotion, I recognize it as a work of art...it is useless for the critic to tell me that something is a work of art; he must make me feel it for myself. This he can do only by making me see; he must get at my emotions through my eyes.[3]

Criticism goes beyond what is seen or heard. It strives to probe and explore the emotional process provoked by the sounds and images. The critic is hopefully capable of sensing and describing that nuance of the work which produces the aesthetic reaction so that the less perceptive and less sensitive person may perceive it and be enriched.

An important requirement for a critic is an unbiased attitude, to be neither protagonist nor antagonist of a specific style, historical period, school of art, or an artist, to keep the artist and work of art separate. Each work of art, visual or otherwise, must be discussed on its own merits. To be unbiased demands a degree of detachment, a stepping away from preconceived parameters. Bias distorts artistic criticism. As Hume expressed it:

> a critic must preserve his mind free from all prejudice, and allow nothing to enter into his consideration but the very object which is submitted to his examination...prejudice is destructive of sound judgement, and prevents all operations of the intellectual faculties.[4]

An unbiased, open, and flexible attitude is not constrained by the demand that the work reflect the temper of the times. Art, regardless of genre, need not fall into the mold of presentness to be worthy of greatness. The narrow critic, frequently deprecates art done in an older manner as if a newly discovered etching by Rembrandt or symphony by Beethoven would be meaningless at this time. The demand that work fall within the modern idiom places an unnecessary constraint upon the artist and forces the artist to consciously or unconsciously work without strong artistic motivation. James Ackerman comments:

> A premium is placed on any sort of change in art, as it is in the design of automobiles and refrigerators. I call this the following of the avant

> garde…the objective of creative activity is the work of art itself, and not any distant goal.[5]

Fads and fashion are all too prevalent in the arts. Occasionally, changes in methodology appear upon the art scene with great rapidity. These changes may be ascribed to a sincere desire to express concepts in a totally new way or else to experiment, but many of these changes are due to the difficulty of advancing aesthetically along the pathways that preceding artists have traveled. It is difficult to outdo Michelangelo, Picasso, or Mozart, or to even stand near them. Such movements, although valid experimentally, may, in the minds of the naive, assume aspects of aesthetic validity much beyond the true nature of the experiment. This does not imply that an experimental statement is necessarily devoid of aesthetic significance. On the contrary, an experimental statement may have as much aesthetic validity as any preceding creative effort regardless of its style or period.

It is irrelevant aesthetically whether a statement is made using an ancient or modern approach. The total end result detached as much as possible from its creator and its historical tie should be the basis of the aesthetic evaluation. The idea of "old fashioned" in art is one of the greatest fallacies in art criticism.

Critics are often inclined to evaluate the aesthetic aspect of the work against some standard. In this respect we must appreciate that to measure aesthetic achievements with any degree of certainty is not possible. Measurement as we know it in physics cannot be applied to the world of music, painting, or the dramatic arts, but lack of a precise measuring-stick does not mean that aesthetic evaluations are meaningless and valueless. It does imply, however, that such evaluations demand extreme caution and restraint.

The critic moves alongside the scholar who may describe various aspects of the art work from the historical to the technical. Sensitivity as to the aesthetic qualities of art is not demanded of the scholar but is demanded of the critic. The critic should be sensitive enough to recognize the emotional impact of a bent wrist or head tilt that may accentuate the sculptural impact or to hear the minor chord interposed in a major-mode work that suddenly alters the sensation aroused by the music. In other words, the critic should have the ability to discern the aspect of the work that makes it art rather than decoration, and should be poet enough to express or explain that Gestalt to perceivers so they may learn how to see, hear, and feel its significance. It is quite rare to encounter a critic capable of doing this. All too often critics lack the sensitivity to perceive adequately or the ability to express feelings. The inability to accomplish this edifying task is the greatest deficit among most art critics.

We can again examine Pinchas Noy's comment concerning Mozart, that portrays how a critic may significantly enhance the joy of listening to music.

> The fourth movement of Mozart's Jupiter symphony…[is] built on five different themes….You can enjoy listening to…nothing more than the single melodic line and its rhythmical beats….But you may receive an even greater pleasure by following various ingenious combinations of two, three or four themes and the inversions from beginning to end…you will achieve greatest pleasure of all if you succeed to follow all five melodic lines of the symphony to their climax…where they converge into a magnificent five-part counterpointal structure.[6]

An outstanding example of the rare critic of visual art is reflected in André Malraux's critique of the artist Georges de La Tour in which he exposes the unique quality that permeates most of his work.

The painting "Magdalen With the Smoking Flame" is quite typical of de La Tour's art. This painting portrays a sense of thoughtful quietness, a reaction to be expected if exposed to the actual scene. But on further study of the painting, we are suddenly aware of an aura of sculptured silence and a darkness that is exquisitely serene and a motionlessness that, although seemingly distant, is expressed by Malraux as an "elemental stillness." Malraux further explores the feeling that may be gained upon study of Georges de La Tour's work.

> La Tour's light creates an all pervasive harmony, an atmosphere of otherworldly calm….La Tour does not paint shadowy backgrounds; he paints night itself…his figures are not isolated from this darkness; rather they are its very emanation….La Tour alone is the interpreter of the serenity that dwells in the heart of darkness…his candle is the source of a diffused light, far from being realistic, is timeless….[7]

There is a monumental, and yet weightless quality in La Tour's figures that is gained through a sense of translucency; all of which conveys an ethereal quality.

These nuances induce an unexpected quality of awe in a moment of poignant thought. With expressions such as these, the paintings of Georges de La Tour, even to the most unsophisticated and insensitive person, become meaningful visual poems.

For another example of how a critic may enhance the perceiver's appreciation, consider the painting "Woman with Blue Veil" by Picasso.

This painting portrays a standing woman who appears pensive and relaxed. What is it about the painting that makes it so special? We may explain how Picasso achieves the feeling of repose by describing the slight droop of the right hand that suggests the feeling of a relaxed state. This is augmented by the casual asymmetrical sag of the top of her blouse, the resting position of her left hand suspended in her pocket and her distant gaze. This description may help explain how Picasso, or any highly skilled and talented artisan may have achieved the overall effect, but it does not explain why the painting achieves the hoped for *unexpected enhancement*. Where is it, and how is it sensed?

Despite the obvious sense of pensive repose that is easily appreciated, further study reveals an element of indecision, a thoughtfulness that is disturbed. This enhancement is gained by the strange placement of the right forearm. It does not simply hang by her side, it is held at waist level suggesting an unconscious plea for help during the pensive state. An unexpected element of pensive indecision occurs. The ability of Picasso to express this subtle unexpected nuance reveals why Picasso is a "real" artist as well as a superb artisan.

James Ackerman comments that:

> Criticism becomes art when it communicates experiences and stimulates sensations that the reader cannot get by himself, just as a still life painting becomes art when it transforms a certain number of apples and bottles into a meaningful formulation of the painter's imagination.[8]

The critic should be dispassionate enough to recognize the aesthetic value of a work of art even though it may not have been a

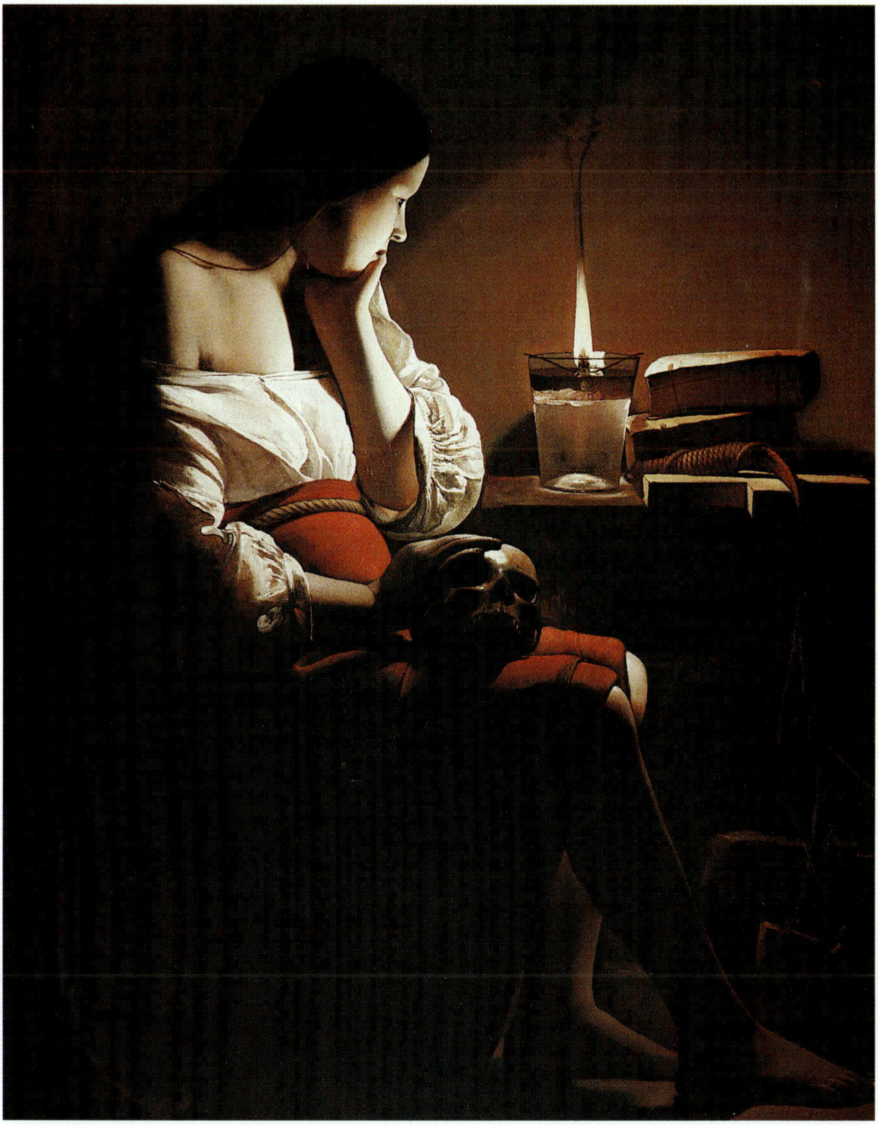

Georges de La Tour, "Magdalen with the Smoking Flame,"[7] reprinted with permission of the Los Angeles County Museum of Art.

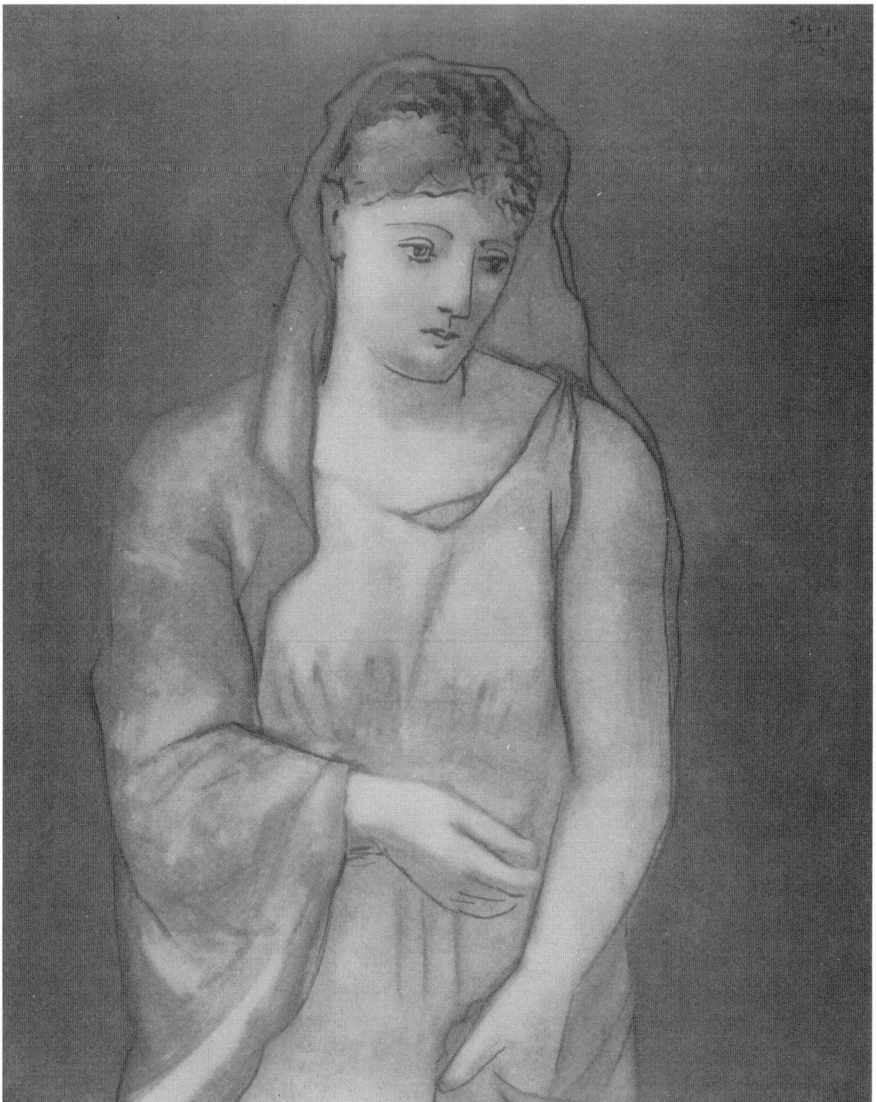

Pablo Picasso, "Woman with Blue Veil," reprinted with permission of the Los Angeles County Museum of Art.

source of pleasure to that individual. Critics may be disturbed by a modern musical composition or a Goya etching, and they may dislike the work, but they should be able to discern qualities in the work that could produce significant aesthetic reactions in others.

Although judgmental elements occur in the evaluation of a work of art, it is unfortunate when that judgment is used to deprecate the aesthetic aspect of the work of a sincere artist. The critic is certainly free to deprecate a play, painting, or musical performance if he or she is able to describe the reasons for condemnation, to elucidate those factors lacking in the work, but discussions that cast blanket condemnation upon sincere creative attempts without clarification are rarely if ever warranted. If the critic is unmoved or uninspired, the critic should discuss those feelings with the realization that what may appear to be an aesthetic desert to the critic may be of aesthetic significance to someone else. If the work lacks aesthetic significance, it will be readily sensed by the public.

Prior to a critic's condemnation of a work of art, he or she should recall that El Greco thought that Michelangelo did not know how to paint; Goethe thought that Dante's *Divine Comedy* was mediocre, T.S. Eliot felt that *Hamlet* was a failure, Whistler remarked that a ten-year-old child could paint as well as Paul Cézanne, and Johann Sebastian Bach was considered a fuddy-duddy and hopelessly old-fashioned.[9] This litany of judgments that did not stand the test of time should be stamped on the walls of all reviewers of the arts.

Critics can contribute significantly to the public. First they can provide the impetus for some perceivers to restudy work of art critiqued to better understand the validity or lack of validity of the critic's comments. Second value lies in the ability of some critics to enable the public to view works of art with an open mind and begin to appreciate new trends in art. In the realm of poetry, where metaphor plays such an important role, the subtleties of the poetic expression may not be readily recognized by the reader even after repeated readings. In this area of the arts, the critic may be of great value to help clarify the meaning of a word that may have been in common use in the distant past or may have been used as a symbol in ancient times. The critic may be able to expose nuances within the poem and to illuminate the intent of the poet through the use of other metaphors or stories that help the reader grasp the deeper meaning of the poem.

As the critic must be cautious and discerning, so must the reader. Critics may obfuscate as well as clarify the significance of words and the poet's intention. The words of the poet, which usually speak for themselves, are often given a different life by the critic with the intent to find a hidden or more subtle thought he or she assumes was in the poet's mind, when in actuality the words mean exactly what the poet wished to express. Poets are usually careful and selective in determining which words are to be used. The critic's interpretation may reflect the critic's psyche more than the poet's intention.

In the realm of music, to appreciate the critic's notes we should listen to the music immediately after reading or hearing the critique. If you had the privilege of hearing Leonard Bernstein's discussion of symphonies or a violinist discuss Vivaldi's "Four Seasons" and then immediately play a rendition of it, you would be aware of nuances within the music that you would otherwise have not noticed.

The interaction of factors forming the aesthetic sense is sufficiently intricate to support a greater restraint in the appraisal of creative deeds by the critic and a greater degree of skepticism by the public in accepting evaluations of the various art forms.

The public is generally reticent to express opinions in areas where they do not have expertise. This is especially true if the element of talent, rather than knowledge, plays a key role. As a result, it is unfortunately prone to accept without much question the opinions about art from the more vociferous, knowledgeable, or talented individuals as valid since they may speak with an aura of authority. A place does exist for connoisseurship, but not for the elitism often seen with it. The expert is not always right, though to be reticent in accepting the opinion of so-called authority does not mean that we should ignore it.

I conclude by recalling, approvingly, Stephen C. Pepper's statement, "An understanding spectator is a critic, and a critic is simply an understanding spectator who is perhaps a little more articulate in communicating the experiences he has in a work."[10]

Notes

Introduction

1. Mary Mothersill, *Beauty Restored* (Oxford: Clarendon Press,1984), pp. 10–12.

2. Morris Weitz, "The Role of Theory in Aesthetics," *The Journal of Aesthetics and Art Criticism* (Summer 1956), p. 27.

3. Susanne K. Langer, *Mind, An Essay on Human Nature* (Baltimore: John Hopkins University Press, 1967), p. 84.

4. Jean Piaget, *Six Psychological Studies*, translated by Anita Tenzer (New York: Random House, 1967), p. 15.

5. Deryck Cooke, *The Language of Music* (Oxford: Oxford University Press, 1989), p. 272.

6. A.J. Ayer, *Language, Truth, and Logic* (London: 1936), quoted by Hugo Meynell in *The Nature of Aesthetic Value* (London: Macmillan Press Ltd., 1986), p. 3.

7. Clive Bell, *Art* (New York: Capricorn Books, G.P. Putnam's Sons, 1958), pp. 16–17.

8. Roger Fry, "Transformations" in E.F. Carritt, *Philosophies of Beauty* (Oxford: The Clarendon Press, 1962), p. 267.

9. H. Kohut and S. Lavarie, "On the Enjoyment of Listening to Music," *Psychoanalytical Quarterly*, 19 (1950), pp. 64–87, p. 67. Pinchus Noy, "Why Do We Enjoy Art?", *Israel Journal of Psychiatry*, 26 (1989), pp. 124–137.

10. Edmund Burke, "A Philosophical Enquiry into the Origin of Our Ideas of the Sublime and the Beautiful" in Burke's *Enquiry into the Sublime and the Beautiful*, ed. J.T. Boulton (London: Routledge and Kegan Paul, 1958), p. 53.

11. Jerome Kagan, *Three Seductive Ideas* (Cambridge, Mass. Harvard University Press, 1998), pp. 151–193, and personal communication, September 2000.

Chapter 1
The Anatomy of Human Emotion

1. James W. Papez, "A Proposed Mechanism of Emotion" *Archives of Neurology and Psychiatry*, 38 (1937), pp. 725–743, p. 726.

2. C.J. Herrick, "The Function of the Olfactory Parts of the Cerebral Cortex," *Proceedings of the National Academy of Science*, 19 (1933), pp. 7–14, p. 8.

3. Paul D. MacLean, "Psychosomatic Disease and the Visceral Brain," *Psychosomatic Medicine*, 11:6 (November-December 1949), pp. 338–353, p. 351.

4. D.W. Ploog and Paul D. MacLean, "Display of Penile Erection in Squirrel Monkey," *Animal Behavior*, 11 (1963) pp. 32–39, p. 35.

5. George Mandler, "The Search for Emotion," in *Emotions: Their Parameters and Measurements*, ed. L. Levi (New York: Raven Press, 1975), pp. 1–15, p. 2.

6. William James, "What Is Emotion?", *Mind*, 9 (1884), pp. 188–205. Walter B. Cannon, "The James Lange Theory of Emotion," *American Journal of Psychology*, 39 (1926), pp. 106–124, p. 107.

7. Paul D. MacLean and D.V. Ploog, "Cerebral Representation of Penile Erection," *Journal of Neurophysiology*, 25 (1962), pp. 29–55, p. 47.

8. M.P. Bishop, S.T. Elder, and R.G. Heath, "Intracranial Self-Stimulation in Man," *Science*, 140 (1963), pp. 393–396, p. 394.

9. Paul D. MacLean, "The Limbic System With Respect to Self-Preservation and the Preservation of the Species," *Journal of Nervous and Mental Disease*, 127 (1958), pp. 1–11.

10. Birger R. Kaada, "Somato-Motor, Autonomic, and Electro-corticographic Responses to Electrical Stimulation of Rhinencephalic and Other Structures in Primates, Cat, and Dog," *Acta Physiologica Scandinavia*, 24 Supplement 83 (1971), pp. 11–285.

11. Walle H.J. Nauta, "The Problem of the Frontal Lobe: A Reinterpretation," *Journal of Psychiatric Research*, 8 (1971), pp. 167–187, p. 182.

Chapter 2
Basic Psychological Mechanisms

1. Austin H. Riesen, "Sensory Deprivation" in *Progress in Physiological Psychology*, ed. B. Stellar and J. Sprague (New York: Academic Press, 1966), pp. 117–147, pp. 140–141.

2. *Ibid.*, pp. 125–126.

3. M.R. Rosenzweig and E.L. Bennet, "Cerebral Effects of Environmental Complexity and Training Among Adults Rats," *Journal of Comparative Physiological Psychology*, 57 (1963), pp. 438–439.

4. Joseph Addison, "The Pleasures of the Imagination," *The Spectator* no. 412, *The Works of Joseph Addison* (New York: G.P. Putnam & Co., 1854), vol. 5, p. 328.

5. Aristotle, *Poetics*, Translated by S.H. Butcher in *A Modern Book of Esthetics*, ed. Melvin Rader (New York: Holt Rinehart and Winston, 1961), bk. 4, p. 488.

6. Paul Eckman and Dacher Keltner, "Universal Facial Expressions of Emotion" in *Nonverbal Communication*, eds. Ullica Segerstrale and Peter Molnar (Mahwah, N.J.: Lawrence Erlbaum Associates, 1997), pp. 34–37.

7. George S. Klein, *Psychoanalytic Theory* (New York: International Universities Press, Inc., 1976), p. 218.

8. Harry F. Harlow, Philip Plubell, and Craig Baysinger, "Induction of Psychological Death in Rhesus Monkeys," *Journal of Autism and Childhood Schizophrenia*, 3:4 (1973), pp. 299–307, p. 302.

9. Paul D. MacLean, "New Findings Relevant to the Evolution of the Psychosexual Functions of the Brain," *Journal of Nervous and Mental Disease*, 135:4 (October 1962), pp. 289–301, p. 295.

10. Sigmund Freud, *Three Contributions to the Theory of Sex*, 4th ed., translated by A.A. Brill (New York: Nervous and Mental Disease Monograph, 1948), pp. 62–63.

11. *Ibid.*, p. 62.

12. D.W. Ploog and Paul .D. MacLean, "Display of Penile Erection in Squirrel Monkey," *Animal Behavior*, 11 (1963), pp. 32–39.

13. *Ibid.*, p. 37.

14. MacLean, "New Findings," p. 299.

15. John Bowlby, *Attachment and Loss* (New York: Basic Books Inc., 1969), vol. 1, pp. 131–132.

16. *Ibid.*, p. 40.

Chapter 3
Emotion and Its Relationship to the Arts

1. Sigmund Freud, "The Moses of Michelangelo" in *Complete Psychological Works of Sigmund Freud*, Standard Edition (London: Hogarth Press, 1955), 13, pp. 209–236, p. 211.

2. Jerome Kagan, personal communication, September 2000.

3. Frank A. Brown Jr., "The Rhythmic Nature of Animals and Plants," *American Scientist*, 47 (June 1959), p. 149.

4. Max Schoen, *The Effects of Music*, ed. Max Schoen (Freeport, N.Y.: Books for Libraries Press, 1968), p. 115.

5. Carl E. Seashore, *Psychology of Music* (New York: Dover Publications Inc., 1967), p. 145.

6. W. Bardas, "Zur Problematik der Musik," *Imago* (1919), 5, pp. 271–364, translated by Pinchas Noy in "The Psycho-dynamic Meaning of Music," Part II, *Journal of Music Therapy*, 4:1 (March 1967), pp. 7–23, p. 20.

7. Dylan Thomas, "Poetic Manifesto," *Texas Quarterly*, 4 (1961), pp. 144–153, p. 125.

8. George Steiner, *Real Presences* (Chicago: The University of Chicago Press, 1991), p. 9.

9. Pinchas Noy, "Why Do We Enjoy Art?", *Israel Journal of Psychiatry*, 26 (1989), pp. 124–137, p. 130.

10. Andrew Cecil Bradley, "Poetry for Poetry's Sake," in A *Modern Book of Esthetics*, 3rd edition, ed. Melvin Rader (New York: Holt Rinehart and Winston, 1961), p. 322.

11. Noy, "Why Do We Enjoy Art?", p. 132.

12. Charles S. Myers in Schoen, *The Effects of Music*, p. 182.

13. C.V. Ramana, "Observations on the Analysis of a Musician," *Samiska*, 6 (1952), pp. 229–242, p. 240. Quoted by Noy, "The Psychodynamic Meaning of Music," p. 84.

14. Max Schoen, "The Aesthetic Attitude in Music," *Psychology Monographs*, 39 (1928), pp. 162–183, p. 182.

15. Peter Kivy, *Sound Sentiment: An Essay on the Musical Emotions, Including the Complete Text of the Corded Shell* (Philadelphia: Temple University Press, 1989), pp. 69–70.

16. Steiner, *Real Presences*, p. 79.

17. Walter J. Dowling and Dane G. Harwood, *Music Cognition* (New York: Academic Press, 1986), p. 208.

18. Marianne Kastner and Robert Crowder, "Perception of the Major/Minor Distinction," *Music Perception*, 8:2 (Winter 1990), pp. 189–202, p. 189.

19. Hermann Helmholtz, *On the Sensations of Tone* (New York: Dover Publications Inc., 1954), p. 216.

20. Deryck Cooke, *The Language of Music* (Oxford: University Press, 1989), p. 57.

21. *Ibid.*, pp. 162–163.

22. C.W. Valentine, "The Aesthetic Appreciation of Musical Intervals Among School Children and Adults," *The British Journal of Psychiatry*, 6 (1913–1914), pp. 190–216, pp. 197–198.

23. Christian P. Heinlein, "The Affective Characters of the Major and Minor Modes in Music," *The Journal of Comparative Psychology*, 8:2 (April 1928), pp. 101–142, p. 140.

24. Robert Crowder, "Perception of the Major/Minor Distinction, Historical and Theoretical Foundations," *Psycho-musicology* 1984, 4:1 and 2, pp. 3–10, p. 5.

25. Johan Sundberg, "Speech, Song, and Emotions," in Manfred Clynes, *Music, Mind, and Brain* (New York: Plenum Press, 1982), pp. 137–149, p. 143.

26. Clynes, *Music, Mind, and Brain*, p. 74.

27. Margarita Mazo, "Lament Made Visible" in *Themes and Variations*, eds. Bell Yung and Joseph S.C. Lam (Cambridge, Mass.: Harvard University Press, 1994), pp. 164–211, pp. 194–202.

28. Margaret Washburn, in Schoen, *The Aesthetic Attitude in Music*, p. 121.

29. Joseph Addison, *The Works of Addison*, 5 (New York: G.P. Putnam & Co., 1854), p. 358.

30. Max Dessoir, *Aesthetics and Theory of Art* (Detroit: Wayne State University Press, 1970), p. 163.

31. Susanne K. Langer, *Feeling and Form* (New York: Charles Scribner's Sons, 1953), p. 405.

32. Aristotle, "On Poetics" *Great Books of the Western World* (Chicago: Encyclopedia Britannica, 1952), 9, ch. 6, p. 684.

33. *American Heritage Dictionary*, ed. William Morris (Boston; Houghton Mifflin Company, 1979).

34. George Santayana, *The Sense of Beauty* (New York: Collier Books, 1961), p. 155.

35. Yrjo Hirn, "Art the Reliever" in Rader, *A Modern Book of Esthetics*, pp. 72–73.

36. Rader, *A Modern Book of Esthetics*, p. xxxii.

37. Joseph Addison, "The Spectator" no. 418, *The Works of Joseph Addison* (Gainesville, Fla.: Scholars' Facsimiles & Reprints, 1963), pp. 359–360.

38. Edward Bullough, "'Psychical Distance'" and a Factor in Art and an Esthetic Principle," in Rader, *A Modern Book of Esthetics*, pp. 394–395.

39. *Ibid*.

40. Edmund Burke, *Enquiry into the Sublime and the Beautiful*, ed. J.T. Boulton (London: Routledge & Kegan Paul, 1958), p. 36.

Chapter 4
A Definition of Aesthetics

1. Wladyslaw Tatarkiewicz, *History of Aesthetics* (The Hague: Mouton Publishers, 1970–1974), p. 292.

2. Alexander G. Baumgarten, in Benedetto Croce, *Aesthetic*, translation by Douglas Ainslie (New York: The Noonday Press, Farrar Strauss & Co., 1962), pp. 212–219, p. 212.

3. Clive Bell, *Art* (New York: Capricorn Books, 1958), p. 17.

4. *Ibid*., p. 22.

5. Theodor Adorno, *Aesthetic Theory*, trans. by C. Lenhardt (London: Routledge & Kegan Paul, 1984), p. 203.

6. Susanne K. Langer, *Feeling and Form* (New York: Charles Scribner's Sons, 1953), pp. 24, 39.

7. William Carlos Williams, *Selected Poems*, edited by Charles Tomlinson (New York: New Direction Books, 1985), p. 125.

8. Glen Wilson, J. Ausman, and T.R. Mathews, "Conservatism and Art Preferences," *Journal of Personality and Social Psychology*, 25:2 (1973), pp. 286–288, p. 288.

9. Hugo A. Meynell, *The Nature of Aesthetic Value* (London: Macmillan Press Ltd., 1986), p. 23.

10. Joseph Addison, *The Works of Addison*, vol. 5, no. 412 (New York: G.P. Putnam & Co.,1854), p. 328.

Chapter 5
Definition of Art

1. Morris Weitz, "The Role of Theory in Aesthetics," *The Journal of Aesthetics and Art Criticism* (Summer 1956), p. 31.

2. Nelson Goodman, "When Is Art?", in *Art and Its Significance*, ed. Stephen Ross (New York: State University of New York Press, 1994), pp. 238–246, p. 245.

3. Erwin Panofsky, *Meaning in the Visual Arts* (Garden City, N.Y.: Doubleday Anchor Books, 1955), p. 14.

4. John Dewey, "Art as Experience," in *Art and Its Significance*, ed. Ross, p. 204.

5. Stephen Pepper, "Organistic Criticism" in Melvin Rader, *A Modern Book of Esthetics* (New York: Holt, Rinehart and Winston, 1961), p. 469.

6. John Hospers, "Problems of Aesthetics," *The Encyclopedia of Philosophy*, vol. 1–2, (New York: Macmillan Publishing Co., Inc, and The Free Press, reprint edition, 1972), pp. 35–56, p. 52.

7. Leo Tolstoy, *What Is Art?* translated by Aylmer Maude (London: Oxford University Press, 1959), p. 123.

8. Vincent Van Gogh, *The Complete Letters of Vincent Van Gogh* (Boston: New York Geographic Society, 1958), 2, Letter 406, p. 375.

9. *Ibid.*, 2, Letter 309, p. 105.

10. Theodor Adorno, *Aesthetic Theory*, trans. by C. Lenhardt (London: Routledge, Kegan Paul, 1984), p. 121.

11. Goodman, "When Is Art?" in *Art and Its Significance*, ed. Ross, p. 244.

12. Van Gogh, *The Complete Letters*, 1, Letter 130, p. 189.

13. Beethoven, quoted by Susanne K. Langer in *Feeling and Form* (New York: Charles Scribner's Sons, 1953), p. 131.

14. Rader, *A Modern Book of Esthetics*, p. xxxi.

15. George Steiner, *Real Presences* (Chicago: The University of Chicago Press, 1991), pp. 216, 228–229.

Chapter 6
The Beautiful, the Sublime, and the Ugly

1. *The Hippias Major*, attributed to Plato, translated by Dorothy Tarrant (New York: Arno Press, 1976), p. xxxi.

2. Jerome Stolnitz, "Beauty: Some Stages in the History of an Idea," *Journal of the History of Ideas*, 22: 2 (April 1961), pp. 185–204, p. 185.

3. Harold Newton Lee, *Perception and Aesthetic Value* (New York: Prentice-Hall, Inc., 1938), pp. 97–98.

4. Theodor Adorno, *Aesthetic Theory*, trans. by C. Lenhardt (London: Routledge & Kegan Paul, 1984), p. 75.

5. Monroe Beardsley, "Plato," *The Encyclopedia of Philosophy* ed. Paul Edwards (New York: Macmillan Pub. Co., 1967), vol. 5–6, p. 19.

6. Francis Hutcheson, *An Inquiry into the Original of Our Ideas of Beauty and Virtue* (1725, 4th ed. London: 1738; Westmead, England: republished by Gregg International Publishers, Ltd., 1969), pp. 14–15.

7. Archibald Alison, *Essays on the Nature and Principles of Taste*, 1790, 4th Ed. (Edinburgh: G. Ramsay for A. Constable, 1815), 1, p. 316.

8. Edmund Burke, *A Philosophical Enquiry into the Origin of Our Ideas of the Sublime and Beautiful*, 1757, ed. J.T. Boulton (London: Routledge and Kegan Paul, 1958), p. 15.

9. Immanuel Kant, *The Critique of Aesthetic Judgment*, in *The Great Books of the Western World*, 42, ed. Robert Maynard Hutchins (Chicago: Encyclopedia Britannica, Inc.,1952), p. 479.

10. Albert Schweitzer, *J.S.Bach*, translated by Ernest Newman (New York: Macmillan Co., 1950), vol. 2, p. 40.

11. Carrol C. Pratt, "Music as the Language of Emotion," A Lecture. The Library of Congress (Washington, 1952), pp. 1–26, p. 26.

12. Max Schoen, *The Effects of Music*, ed. Max Schoen (Freeport, N.Y.: Books for Libraries Press, 1968), pp. 131, 151.

13. *Oxford English Dictionary* (Oxford: Oxford University Press, 1971).

14. Susanne K. Langer, *Feeling and Form* (New York: Charles Scribner's Sons, 1953), p. 396.

15. Burke, *A Philosophical Enquiry*, p. 92.

16. Kant, *The Critique of Aesthetic Judgment*, p. 478.

17. Frans Hemsterhuis, quoted in Leo Tolstoy, *What Is Art?* (London: Oxford University Press, 1959), p. 96.

18. Sigmund Freud, "Civilization and Its Discontents" in *Great Books of the Western World*, 54, ed. Hutchins, p. 775.

19. Guy Sircello, *A New Theory of Beauty* (Princeton: Princeton University Press, 1975), p. 138.

20. *Oxford English Dictionary* (Oxford: Oxford University Press, 1971). *Webster's New International Dictionary*, 2nd ed. unabridged (Springfield, Mass: G & C Merriam Co., 1947). *American Heritage Dictionary* ed. William Morris (Boston: Houghton Mifflin Co., 1979).

21. George Santayana, *The Sense of Beauty* (New York: Collier Books, 1961), p. 167.

22. Bendetto Croce, *Aesthetic* (New York: Noonday Press, 1922), p. 90.

23. Robin G. Collingwood "Outlines of a Philosophy of Art," in E.F. Carritt, *Philosophies of Beauty* (Oxford: Clarendon Press, 1962), p. 293.

24. Burke, *A Philosophical Enquiry*, pp. 113–114, p. 58.

25. Croce, *Aesthetic*, p. 343.

26. Burke, *A Philosophical Enquiry*, p. 51.

27. Alexander Gerard, *An Essay on Taste* (Gainesville, Fla.: Scholars' Facsimiles & Reprints, 1963), pp. 11–29, p. 11.

28. Kant, *Critique of Aesthetic Judgment*, Para. 23.

29. Jerome Stolnitz, "Ugliness," *The Encyclopedia of Philosophy*, 8, ed. Paul Edwards (New York: Macmillan Publishing Co., Inc. and The Free Press, 1967), reprint edition. 1972), vol. 7–8, p. 174.

30. James L. Jarrett, *The Quest for Beauty* (Englewood Cliffs, N. J.: Prentice Hall Inc., 1962), p. 274.

31. Burke, *A Philosophical Enquiry*, p. 119.

Chapter 7
Psychological Aspects of Non-Objective Art

1. Piet Mondrian, "Plastic Art and Pure Plastic Art" in *Art and Its Significance*, ed. Stephen Ross (New York: State University of New York Press, 1994), pp. 677–690, p. 684.

2. Ibid, pp. 682–687.

3. Joseph Addison, "The Spectator," in *The Works of Joseph Addison*, (New York: G.P. Putnam & Co., 1854), 5: No. 411, p. 323.

4. James C. Ackerman, "Abstract Art and the Critics," *The Atlantic Monthly*, 210 (October 1962), pp. 73–78, p. 75.

Chapter 8
The Artist, the Perceiver, and the Aesthetic Lens

1. J.W.N. Sullivan, *The Limitations of Science* (New York: Mentor Books, 1949), p. 117.

2. Benedetto Croce, "Intuition and Expression," in *A Modern Book of Esthetics*, ed. Melvin Rader (New York: Holt, Rinehart and Winston, 1961), p. 103.

3. Vincent Van Gogh, *The Complete Letters of Vincent Van Gogh* (Boston: New York Graphic Society, 1958), 1, Letter no.130, p. 189; Letter no. 257, p. 520.

4. Roger Fry, *Vision and Design* (London: Pelican Books, The Whitefriars Press Ltd., 1961), p. 230.

5. John Dewey, "Art as Experience," in *Art and Its Significance* ed. Stephen Ross New York: State University of New York Press, 1994), p. 208.

6. Richard Strauss, quoted by John Hospers, "The Problems of Aesthetics," *The Encyclopedia of Philosophy*, 1, ed. Paul Edwards (New York: Macmillan Publishing Co., Inc. and The Free Press, 1967), p. 47.

7. Thomas Carlyle, *On Heroes and Hero Worship* (London: Oxford University Press, 1950), p. 122.

8. Martin Heidegger, "The Origin of the Work of Art," in Ross, *Art and Its Significance*, p. 274.

9. Clive Bell, *Art* (New York: Capricorn Books, 1958), p. 19.

10. Hugo A. Meynell, *The Nature of Aesthetic Value* (London: Macmillan Press Ltd., 1986), p. 22.

11. See David E.W. Fenner, *The Aesthetic Attitude* (Atlantic Highlands, N.J., Humanities Press, 1996).

12. Roger Fry, *Vision and Design* (London: Pelican Books, The Whitefriars Press Ltd., 1961), p. 29.

13. George Steiner, *Real Presences* (Chicago: The University of Chicago Press, 1991), p. 9.

14. William Blake, "Auguries of Innocence," *The Harvard Classics*, 41, ed. Charles W. Elliot (New York: P.P. Collier & Sons Co., 1910), p. 106.

Chapter 9
Obligations Between the Artist and Society

1. Vincent Van Gogh, *The Complete Letters of Vincent Van Gogh* (Boston: New York Graphic Society, 1958), 2, Letter no. B19, p. 517.

2. James Jarrett, *The Quest for Beauty* (Englewood Cliffs, N.J.: Prentice Hall Inc., 1962), p. 277.

3. Bell, Clive, *Art* (New York: Capricorn Books, 1958), p. 167.

Chapter 10
The Critic

1. Homer, *The Iliad* (Baltimore: Penguin Books, 1965), pp. 349–350.

2. George Steiner, *Real Presences* (Chicago: The University of Chicago Press, 1991), p. 8.

3. Clive Bell, *Art* (New York: Capricorn Books, 1958), pp. 16–18.

4. David Hume "Of the Standard of Taste" in Melvin Rader, *A Modern Book of Aesthetics* (New York: Holt, Rinehart and Winston, 1961), pp. 456–457.

5. James C. Ackerman, "Art History and the Problems of Criticism," *Daedalus* (Winter 1960), pp. 253–263, p. 259.

6. Noy, Pinchas, "Why Do We Enjoy Art?", *Israel Journal of Psychiatry,* 26 (1989), pp. 124–137, p. 132.

7. André Malraux, *The Voices of Silence* (Garden City, N.Y.: Doubleday and Co. Inc., 1953), pp. 390–396.

8. Ackerman, "Art History and the Problems of Criticisms," p .254.

9. James Jarrett, *The Quest for Beauty* (Englewood Cliffs, N.J.: Prentice Hall Inc., 1962), p. 260.

10. Stephen C. Pepper, "Organistic Criticism," in Rader, *A Modern Book of Aesthetics,* p. 475.

Bibliography

Ackerman, James. "Abstract Art and the Critics," *The Atlantic Monthly*, 210 (October 1962), pp. 73–78.

———. "Art History and the Problems of Criticism," *Daedalus* (Winter 1960), pp. 253–263.

Addison, Joseph. *The Works of Joseph Addison*, vol. 5, *The Spectator*, nos. 411, 412, 418, New York: G.P. Putnam & Co., 1854.

Adorno, Theodor. *Aesthetic Theory*, translated by C. Lenhardt. London: Routledge & Kegan Paul, 1984.

Alison, Archibald. *Essays on the Nature and Principles of Taste*. 1790, 4th ed. Edinburgh: G Ramsay for A. Constable, 1815.

Aristotle. *Poetics*, translated by S.H. Butcher in *A Modern Book of Aesthetics*, edited by Melvin Rader. New York: Holt Rinehart and Winston, 1961.

———. *On Poetics, Great Books of the Western World*. Chicago: Encyclopaedia Britannica, Inc. 1952. vol 9.

Ayer, A.J. *Language, Truth, and Logic*. London: 1936, quoted by Hugo A. Meynell in *The Nature of Aesthetic Value*. London: Macmillan Press Ltd., 1986.

Bardas, W. "Zur Problematik der Musik," *Imago*, 5 (1919), 271–364, translated by Pinchas Noy in "The Psychodynamic Meaning of Music," Part 2, *Journal of Music Therapy*, 4:1 (March 1967), pp. 7–23.

Baumgarten, Alexander. In Benedetto Croce, *Aesthetic*, translated by Douglas Ainslie. New York: The Noonday Press, Farrar Strauss & Co., 1962, pp. 212–219.

Beardsley, Monroe. "Plato," *The Encyclopedia of Philosophy*, edited by Paul Edwards. New York: Macmillan Pub. Co., 1967. vol. 5–6.

Bell, Clive. *Art*. New York: Capricorn Books, 1958.

Bishop, M., S.T. Elder, and R.G. Heath. "Intracranial Self-Stimulation in Man," *Science*, 140 (1963), pp. 394–396.

Blake, William. "Auguries of Innocence." *The Harvard Classics* 41, edited by Charles W. Elliot. New York: P.P. Collier & Sons Co., 1910.

Bosanquet, Bernard. *A History of Aesthetic*. New York: Meridian Books, 1957.

———. *Three Lectures on Aesthetic*. London: Macmillan and Company, 1931.

Bowlby, John. *Attachment and Loss*. New York: Basic Books Inc., 1969.

Bradley, Andrew. "Poetry for Poetry's Sake," in *A Modern Book of Aesthetics*, 3rd ed., edited by Melvin Rader. New York: Holt, Rinehart and Winston, 1961.

Brown, Frank A. "The Rhythmic Nature of Animals and Plants, *American Scientist*, 47 (June 1959), pp. 147–168.

Bullough, Edward. "'Psychical Distance' as a Factor in Art and an Esthetic Principle," in Melvin Rader, *A Modern Book of Aesthetics*, 3rd ed. New York: Holt, Rinehart and Winston, 1961.

Burke, Edmund. "A Philosophical Enquiry into the Origin of Our Ideas of the Sublime and Beautiful," in *Burke's Enquiry into the Sublime and Beautiful*, edited by J.T. Boulton. London: Routledge and Kegan Paul, 1958.

Cannon, Walter. "The James-Lange Theory of Emotion." *American Journal of Psychology*, 39 (1926), pp. 86–124.

Carlyle, Thomas. *On Heroes and Hero Worship*. London: Oxford University Press, 1950.

Carritt, E.F. *Philosophies of Beauty*. Oxford: The Clarendon Press, 1962.

Clynes, Manfred. *Music, Mind, and Brain: The Neuro-psychology of Music*. New York: Plenum Press, 1982.

Cooke, Deryck. *The Language of Music*. Oxford: Oxford University Press, 1989.

Croce, Benedetto. *Aesthetic*, translated by Douglas Ainslie. New York: The Noonday Press, Farrar Strauss & Co., 1962.

———. "Intuition and Expression" in *A Modern Book of Esthetics*, edited by Melvin Rader. New York: Holt Rinehart and Winston, 1961.

Crowder, Robert. "Perception of the Major/Minor Distinction: IV. Emotional Connotations in Young Children," *Music Perception*, 8:2 (Winter 1990), pp. 189–202.

Delgado, Jose, Warren W. Roberts, and Neal E. Miller. "Learning Motivated by Electrical Stimulation of the Brain," *American Journal of Physiology*, 179 (1954), pp. 587–592.

Dessoir, Max. *Aesthetics and Theory of Art*. Detroit: Wayne State University Press, 1970.

Dewey, John. "Art as Experience," in *Art and Its Significance*, edited by Stephen Ross. New York: State University of New York Press, 1994.

Dowling, Walter J. and Dane G. Harwood. *Music Cognition*. New York: Academic Press, 1986.

Ekman,Paul and Dacher Keltner. "Universal Facial Expressions of Emotion" in *Nonverbal Communication*, eds. Ullica Segerstrale and Peter Molnar. Mahwah, N.J.: L.E.A Publishers, 1997.

Fenner, David. *The Aesthetic Attitude*. Atlantic Highlands, N.J.: Humanities Press, 1996.

Freud, Sigmund. *Three Contributions to the Theory of Sex*. 4th ed. translated by A.A. Brill. New York: Nervous and Mental Disease Monograph, 1948.

———. "The Moses of Michelangelo," in *Complete Psychological Works of Sigmund Freud*. Standard Edition, 13. London: Hogarth Press, 1955–1956, pp. 209–236.

———. *Civilization and Its Discontents* in *Great Books of the Western World*, vol. 54, edited by Robert M. Hutchins. Chicago: Encyclopedia Britannica, 1952.

Fry, Roger. *Vision and Design*. London: Pelican Books, The Whitefriars Press Ltd., 1961.

Gerard, Alexander. *An Essay on Taste*. Gainesville, Fla: Scholars' Facsimiles Reprints, 1963.

Goodman, Nelson. "When Is Art?", in *Art and Its Significance*, edited by Stephen Ross, New York: State University of New York Press, 1994.

Greene, Theodore. "The Nature and Criteria of Criticism," in Melvin Rader, *A Modern Book of Aesthetics*. New York: Holt, Rinehart and Winston, 1961.

Harlow, Harry, Philip Plubell, and Craig Baysinger. "Induction of Psychological Death in Rhesus Monkeys," *Journal of Autism and Childhood Schizophrenia*, 3:4 (1973), pp. 299–307.

Harwood, Dane. *Music Cognition*. New York: Academic Press, 1986.

Heidegger, Martin. "The Origin of the Work of Art," in *Art and Its Significance*, 3rd ed, edited by Stephen Ross. New York: State University of New York Press, 1994.

Heinlein, Chester. "The Affective Characters of the Major and Minor Modes in Music." *The Journal of Comparative Psychology*. 8:2 (April 1928), pp. 101–142.

Helmholtz, Hermann von. *On the Sensations of Tone*. New York: Dover Publications Inc., 1954.

Hemsterhuis, Frans. quoted in Leo Tolstoy, *What Is Art*? London: Oxford University Press, 1959. translation and quotation from Schasler, *Kritische Geshichte der Aesthetik*. 1872, 1 and 2, pp. 331–333.

Herrick, C. "The Functions of the Olfactory Parts of the Cerebral Cortex." *Proceedings of the National Academy of Science*, 19 (1933), pp. 7–14.

Hirn, Yrjo. "Art the Reliever," in Melvin Rader, *A Modern Book of Aesthetics*. New York: Holt, Rinehart and Winston, 1961.

Homer. *The Iliad*. Baltimore: Penguin Books, 1965.

Hospers, John. "Problems of Aesthetics," *The Encyclopedia of Philosophy*. New York: Macmillan Publishing Co., Inc, and The Free Press, reprint edition, 1972. vol. 1–2.

Hume, David. "Of the Standard of Taste" in Melvin Rader, *A Modern Book of Aesthetics*. New York: Holt, Rinehart and Winston, 1961.

Hutcheson, Francis. *An Inquiry into the Original of Our Ideas of Beauty and Virtue*. 1725, 4th ed. Westmead, England: Gregg International Publishers, Ltd., 1969.

James, William. "What Is Emotion?", *Mind*, 9 (1884), pp. 188–205.

———.*The Principles of Psychology*. New York: H. Holt, 1890.

Jarrett, James. *The Quest for Beauty*. Englewood Cliffs, N.J.: Prentice Hall Inc., 1962.

Kaada, Birger. "Somato-motor, Autonomic, and Electro-Corticographic Responses to Electrical Stimulation of Rhinencephalic' and Other Structures in Primates,

Cat, and Dog," *Acta Physiologica Scandinavia*, 24. (Supplement 83 (1951), pp. 1–285.

Kant, Immanuel. *The Critique of Aesthetic Judgment*, in *The Great Books of the Western World*, 42, edited by Robert Maynard Hutchins. Chicago: Encyclopedia Britannica, Inc., 1952.

Kastner, Marianne. "Perception of the Major/Minor Distinction: IV. Emotional Connotations in Young Children," *Music Perception*, 8:2 (Winter 1990), pp. 189–202.

Kivy, Peter. *Sound Sentiment: An Essay on the Musical Emotions, Including the Complete Text of the Corded Shell*. Philadelphia: Temple University Press, 1989.

Klein, George S. *Psychoanalytic Theory*. New York: International Universities Press, Inc. 1976.

Kohut, H., and S. Levarie. "On the Enjoyment of Listening to Music," *Psychanalytical Quarterly*, 19 (1950), pp. 64–87,

Langer, Susanne K. *Mind: An Essay on Human Nature.* Baltimore: John Hopkins University Press, 1967.

———. *Feeling and Form*. New York: Charles Scribner's Sons 1953.

Lavarie, S. "On the Enjoyment of Listening to Music," *Psychoanalytical Quarterly*, 19 (1950), pp. 64–87.

Lee, Harold. *Perception and Aesthetic Value.* New York: Prentice-Hall, Inc., 1938.

MacLean, Paul and D.V. Ploog. "Cerebral Representation of Penile Erection," *Journal of Neurophysiology*, 25 (1962), pp. 29–55.

———."The Limbic System with Respect to Self-Preservation and the Preservation of the Species," *Journal of Nervous and Mental Disease*, 127 (1958), pp. 1–11.

———."New Findings Relevant to the Evolution of the Psychosexual Functions of the Brain," *Journal of Nervous and Mental Disease*, 135:4 (October 1962), pp. 289–301.

———."Psychosomatic Disease and the Visceral Brain," *Psychosomatic Medicine*, 11:6 (November-December 1949), pp. 338–353.

Malraux, André. *The Voices of Silence.* Garden City, N.Y.: Doubleday and Co. Inc., 1953.

Mandler, George. "The Search for Emotion," in *Emotions: Their Parameters and Measurements*, edited by L. Levi. New York: Raven Press, 1975.

Mazo, Margarita. "Lament Made Visible" in *Themes and Variations*. eds. Bell Yung and Joseph Lam. Cambridge, Mass.: Harvard University Press, 1994, pp. 164–211.

Meynell, Hugo A. *The Nature of Aesthetic Value*. London: Macmillan Press Ltd., 1986.

Mondrian. Piet. "Plastic Art and Pure Plastic Art," in *Art and Its Significance*, edited by Stephen Ross. New York: State University of New York Press, 1994, pp. 677–690.

Mothersill, Mary. *Beauty Restored*. Oxford: Clarendon Press, 1984.

Nauta, Walle. "The Problem of the Frontal Lobe: A Reinterpretation," *Journal of Psychiatric Research*, 8 (1971), pp. 167–187.

Noy, Pinchas. "Why Do We Enjoy Art?" *Israel Journal of Psychiatry*, 26 (1989), pp. 124–137.

———."The Psychodynamic Meaning of Music," Part II, *Journal of Music Therapy*, 4:1 (March 1967), pp. 7–23.

Olds, James and Peter Milner. "Stimulation Studies: Positive Reinforcement Produced by Electrical Stimulation of Septal Area and Other Regions of the Rat Brain." *Journal of Comparative and Physiological Psychology*, 47 (1954), pp. 419–427.

Panofsky, Erwin. *Meaning in the Visual Arts*. Garden City, N.Y.: Doubleday Anchor Books, 1955.

Papez, James. "A Proposed Mechanism of Emotion." *Archives of Neurology and Psychiatry*, 38 (1937), pp. 725–743.

Pepper, Stephen C. "Organistic Criticism" in Melvin Rader, *A Modern Book of Aesthetics*. New York: Holt, Rinehart and Winston, 1961.

Piaget, Jean. *Six Psychological Studies*. translated by A. Tenzer. New York: Random House, 1967.

Plato. *Sophist*, in *Dialogues of Plato*, translated by Benjamin Jowett. *Great Books of the Western World*, 7, edited by Robert Maynard Hutchins. Chicago: Encyclopedia Britannica, 1952.

———. *The Hippias Major*, attributed to Plato, translated by Dorothy Tarrant. New York: Arno Press, 1976.

Ploog, Detlev W. "Display of Penile Erection in Squirrel Monkey (*saimiri sciureus*)," *Animal Behavior*, 11 (1963), pp. 32–39.

Prall, D.W. *Aesthetic Judgement*. New York: Thomas Y. Crowell Co., Apollo edition, 1967.

Pratt, Carroll C. "Music as the Language of Emotion," A Lecture. Washington D. C.: The Library of Congress, 1950, pp. 1–26.

Rader, Melvin. *A Modern Book of Esthetics*. New York: Holt, Rinehart and Winston, 3rd. edition 1961.

Riesen, A. "Sensory Deprivation," in *Progress in Physiological Psychology*, edited by B. Stellar and J. Sprague. New York: Academic Press, 1966, pp. 117–147.

Rosenzweig, M. and E.L. Bennett. "Cerebral Effects of Environmental Complexity and Training Among Adult Rats," *Journal of Comparative Physiological Psychology*, 57 (1963), pp. 438–439.

Ross, Stephen. *Art and Its Significance*, 3rd ed. Albany, N.Y: State University of New York Press, 1994.

Santayana, George. *The Sense of Beauty*. New York: Collier Books, 1961.

Schoen, Max. *The Effects of Music,* edited by Max Schoen. Freeport, N.Y: Books for Libraries Press, 1968.

———."The Aesthetic Attitude in Music," *Psychology Monographs*, 39 (1928), pp. 162–183.

Schweitzer, Albert. *J.S. Bach*. translated by Ernest Newman, 2 vols. New York: Macmillan Co., 1950.

Seashore, Carl. *Psychology of Music*. New York: Dover Publications, Inc., 1967.

Sircello, Guy. *A New Theory of Beauty*. Princeton: Princeton University Press, 1975.

Steiner, George. *Real Presences*. Chicago: The University of Chicago Press, 1991.

Stolnitz, Jerome. "Beauty: Some Stages in the History of an Idea," *Journal of the History of Ideas*, 22:2 (April 1961), pp. 185–204.

Strauss, Richard. quoted by John Hospers, "Problems of Aesthetics," *The Encyclopedia of Philosophy*, 1, edited by Paul Edwards. New York: Macmillan Publishing Co., Inc. and The Free Press, 1967.

Sullivan, J. *The Limitations of Science.* New York: Mentor Books, 1949.

Tatarkiewicz, Wladyslaw. *History of Aesthetics.* The Hague: Mouton Publishers, 1970–1974.

Thomas, Dylan. "Poetic Manifesto," *Texas Quarterly*, 4 (1961), pp. 44–53.

Tolstoy, Leo. *What Is Art?* translated by Aylmer Maude. London: Oxford University Press, 1959.

Valentine, Charles W. "The Aesthetic Appreciation of Musical Intervals Among School Children and Adults," *The British Journal of Psychiatry*, 6 (1913–1914), pp. 190–216.

Van Gogh, Vincent. *The Complete Letters of Vincent Van Gogh.* Boston: New York Graphic Society, 1958.

Washburn, Margaret. "The Aesthetic Attitude in Music," in *The Effects of Music*, edited by Max Schoen. Freeport, New York: Books for Libraries Press, 1968.

Weitz, Morris. "The Role of Theory in Aesthetics," *The Journal of Aesthetics and Art Criticism* (Summer 1956), pp. 27–30.

Williams, William Carlos. *Selected Poems*, edited by Charles Tomlinson. New York: New Directions Books, 1985.

Wilson, Glen, James Ausman, and Thomas R. Mathews. "Conservatism and Art Preferences," *Journal ofPersonality and Social Psychology*, 25:2 (1973), pp. 286–288.

Index

NEW STUDIES IN AESTHETICS

Robert Ginsberg, General Editor

Victor Yelverton Haines & Jo Ellen Jacobs, *Associate Editors*

This series publishes explorative thinking in the philosophy of art as well as in the philosophy of life. Applied aesthetics and theoretical development of non-traditional topics are considered, along with traditional studies in aesthetic theory or the problems specific arts. Well-written volumes may take the form of monographs, treatises, collected essays, proceedings, reference works, and translations. Use of illustrations is encouraged. In addition to works in English, texts in German, French, Spanish, Italian, and other languages may be published.

For additional information about this series or for the submission of manuscripts, please contact:

Peter Lang Publishing, Inc.
Acquisitions Department
516 N. Charles St., 2nd Floor
Baltimore, MD 21201

To order other books in this series, please contact our Customer Service Department:

(800) 770-LANG (within the U.S.)
(212) 647-7706 (outside the U.S.)
(212) 647-7707 FAX